KOSHER MACROS

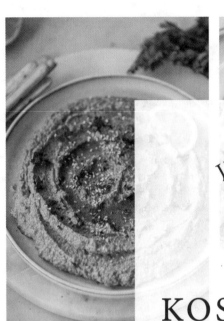
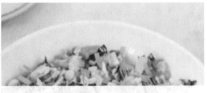
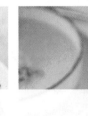

JEWISH FOOD HERO

Nourishing your mind, body, and spirit

—

KOSHER MACROS

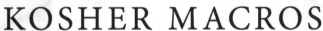

63 Recipes for Eating Everything (Kosher) for
Physical Health and Emotional Balance

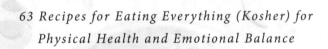

—

Kenden Alfond

Author of *Feeding Women of the Talmud, Feeding Ourselves*

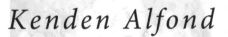

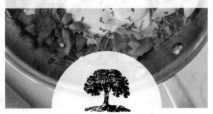

TURNER
PUBLISHING COMPANY

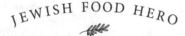

Nourishing your mind, body, and spirit

Kosher Macros: 63 Recipes for Eating Everything (Kosher) for Physical Health and Emotional Balance

TURNER PUBLISHING COMPANY
Nashville, Tennessee
www.turnerpublishing.com

Cover and book design by William Ruoto

Library of Congress Cataloging-in-Publication Data

Names: Alfond, Kenden, author.

Title: Kosher macros : 63 recipes for eating Everything (Kosher) for physical health and emotional balance / Kenden Alfond, author of Feeding Women of the Talmud, Feeding Ourselves.

Description: Nashville, Tennessee : Turner Publishing Company, [2023] | Series: Jewish food hero | Includes index.

Identifiers: LCCN 2023009061 | ISBN 9781684429059 (paperback) | ISBN 9781684429066 (hardcover) | ISBN 9781684429073 (epub)

Subjects: LCSH: Jewish cooking. | Kosher food. | Nutrition. | LCGFT: Cookbooks.

Classification: LCC TX724 .A4454 2023 | DDC 641.5/676—dc23/eng/20230310

LC record available at https://lccn.loc.gov/2023009061

Printed in the United States of America

For my daughter, Yaël

Since maintaining a healthy and sound body is among the ways of God - for one cannot understand or have any knowledge of the Creator, if he is ill - therefore, he must avoid that which harms the body and accustom himself to that which is healthful and helps the body become stronger.[1]

—Maimonides Mishneh Torah, Human Dispositions 4:1[2]

---

[1] Gendered language; This original text uses male-gendered language. We've preserved the original language out of respect to the text, but this quote can easily be read with other pronouns and reclaimed for one's own story.

[2] Trans. by Eliyahu Touger, Moznaim Publishing

CONTENTS

CONTENTS

KOSHER MACROS

INTRODUCTION

STORY

In June 2021, after eating a vegetarian/vegan/plant-based diet for twenty-plus years, I transitioned to eating a kosher omnivore diet. I changed the way I was eating because I was feeling physically unwell, and my exclusive dietary pattern was creating mental and emotional unease for me. As the mother of a child approaching adolescence, I also sensed I needed to make changes in our family food culture.

Food had become a drag for me. My family and I had recently relocated from Cambodia to France, and I longed to regain pleasure and excitement in eating and to enjoy the new ingredients and treats available to me in my new home. I wanted to make the most of sharing food with my family and new friends.

After eating so long within a rigid vegan/vegetarian framework, I had to relearn how to eat in balance, free from food restrictions, obsessions, and deprivation. I was also coming to the slow (and embarrassing) realization that, since my late teens, I had fallen prey to nutrition misinformation, baseless nutrition trends, and sensationalist ideas about food. Being influenced by food fads and misdirected health claims had led me to adopt extreme ideas about food and eating habits—all of which I was keen to leave behind.

I started researching the macros method because it appeared to be a flexible and inclusive way of approaching food—the ideal structure to support me to eat everything (kosher) in balance. So I started on my learning pathway about macros. I went down many rabbit holes of information: I was searching through online recipes and blogs as well as physical recipe books, navigating from one topic to the next. It was overwhelming trying to "digest" the high volume of material available and to decipher which parts were objectively credible. During this initial learning phase I also found that most recipes I came across simply did not meet kosher requirements. To feel "at home" with the macros eating pattern, I needed kosher recipes that resonated with the Jew-ish food landscape.

This all led me to do two things simultaneously over the next eighteen months:

1. Hire nutrition experts to coach me through macros and the transition to eating everything (kosher).
2. Write this book!

This *Kosher Macros* cookbook will:

*   share what I have learned about the macros eating method in plain and easy-to-understand language, so you can implement it with ease at home; and
*   give you sixty-three macros-friendly kosher recipes, which are all simple to make, delicious, and can be enjoyed by anyone, regardless of kosher observance.

WHAT IS A MACROS DIETARY PATTERN?

Macronutrients ("macro" meaning big) refers to the broad food categories: proteins, carbohydrates, and fats. These provide, among other things, fuel for our bodies. A macros dietary pattern is one where a person tracks these three main groups to consume certain proportions and amounts, set according to the calories their body needs every day.

MACRONUTRIENTS AT-A-GLANCE		
CARBS *Energy*	**PROTEIN** *Strength*	**FAT** *Hormonal Balance*
ENERGY: 4 calories per gram **FUNCTIONS:** Carbs are the primary and essential energy source for the body. The body breaks carbs down into glucose, which fuels the cells, tissues, and organs. **RECOMMENDED INTAKE:** 45% - 65%	**ENERGY:** 4 calories per gram **FUNCTIONS:** Proteins are needed for creating, building and repairing cells. Proteins transport nutrients in the body - vitamins, minerals, sugars, cholesterol, oxygen through the circulatory system to cells and tissues to function normally. **RECOMMENDED INTAKE:** 10% - 35%	**ENERGY:** 9 calories per gram **FUNCTIONS:** Fats provide energy and support for cell growth, protects the organs, maintains steady blood pressure and cholesterol, and is needed for vitamin absorption. **RECOMMENDED INTAKE:** 20% - 35%

In order to build the ideal eating plan, calculate your "macros" plan based on specific health goals. Your health goals establish how many calories to eat per day, and how many macros you require each day, based on:

- current physical attributes: sex, weight, height, and age
- daily level of physical activity
- personal health goals to either maintain, increase, or decrease body weight

I've created a worksheet to make calculating your macros easy—see Appendix A: Calculate Your Macros Worksheet on page 167. Use this as a guide, and expect to do a little trial, error, and tweaking to find the macros balance that works best for you.

ABOUT MICRONUTRIENTS

Micronutrients ("micro" meaning small) are vitamins and minerals—essential nutrients that the body needs in order to function. It is best to get micronutrients from whole foods rather than supplements (pills and powders).

Unlike macronutrients, micronutrients are substances that perform essential tasks without delivering energy. They are essential for making the body operate well and for good health. For example, some are involved in essential enzymatic reactions, and others play an antioxidant role.

TRACKING MACROS EXPLAINED

To "track" macros essentially means to keep a daily food record and capture real-time and accurate data about what you are *actually* eating.

The philosophy behind tracking is "measure to manage." Most people have little to no idea about their food portion sizes and how many carbohydrates, proteins, and fats they eat at individual meals or throughout the day. Tracking macros is a way to make yourself aware of what you are really eating, your total calorie intake, and individual micronutrients in order to manage your overall health and body weight skillfully.

Your body is tracking macros all the time even if you are not. Tracking allows you to tailor the quantity and types of foods you eat to meet your daily calorie and macronutrient goals.

Tracking the food you eat every day (for a finite period of time) allows you to learn to eat everything in balance. The act of tracking your food intake day after day makes you more aware of portion sizes. With time and consistency, eating appropriate portions and proportions of macronutrients becomes a habit. This habit is one of the keys to lifelong health and weight management.

Through tracking, you understand how much of each macronutrient (carbohydrate, protein, and fat) you are eating and how it impacts your physique (form, size, and development of your body), internal body functioning, and relationship with food.

While tracking your daily macros, it's beneficial to see the macros goals as five-gram ranges. While tracking, you will see that the daily macros numbers vary and are rarely perfectly aligned with your goal number. Obsessing about getting your macros numbers exactly right is counterproductive. While tracking, especially when you start, focus on meeting your calorie goal and reaching your macronutrient goal for protein first.

Added to this is that your macros numbers will change as you tweak them to reach different health and physique goals and to respond to different stages in your life.

Tracking teaches you how to think about balancing your macros within each meal and snack. It also helps you to understand how to balance your food intake throughout the day: a carb-heavy lunch may lead to a protein-rich dinner, and so on.

After tracking food for a period of time, you stop mentally registering food within supposedly moral categories of "healthy/unhealthy" and "good/bad." Instead, you begin to conceptualize foods more as they "track": simply as sources of protein, fats, or carbohydrates.

Once you let go of moral categorization of food and focus on the macronutrients you are eating, it becomes easier to sustain a balanced lifestyle. This is not a restrictive or obscure diet, so it does not infringe on your ability to relax and enjoy social and family eating situations; you can enjoy the same food as everyone else because you are simply tracking rather than prohibiting food intake. You can adapt your diet to changing environments, which is one key to maintaining a balanced diet and achieving long-term and lasting results.

To someone like me—who enjoys and thrives on structure—this type of systematic approach felt comfortable and exciting. But maybe you are someone who prefers a more flexible and fluid approach to life! If so, by now, you might think that the macros eating pattern is far too much work. But here's the thing: you only need to track macros for a relatively short time in order to habituate yourself to the pattern and thereafter have a more intuitive sense of the foods and portion sizes that allow you to feed yourself well.

To help you get started with tracking, see:

- Appendix B: Tracking Macros: Step-by-Step on page 173
- Appendix C: Tracking: Pro-Tips on page 179

HOW TO FIGURE OUT YOUR MACRONUTRIENT GOAL NUMBER

When you are trying to find your macronutrient goal number, it is helpful to know that there is an established range: the Acceptable Macronutrient Distribution Range (AMDR). These numbers illustrate a range of intakes for all three macronutrients. The ratio of each macronutrient's contribution to the daily calorie total is expressed in percentages.

Carbohydrates: 45%–65% of total daily caloric intake

Protein: 20%–35% of total daily caloric intake

Fat: 10%–35% of total daily caloric intake, limiting saturated and trans fats

However, since we all have different health goals and health issues, we all need to tweak our macros percentages and calories to find the balance point.

See Appendix D: Four Phases of Macros Tracking.

Calculate your macronutrient target numbers using Appendix A: Calculate Your Macros Worksheet on page 167.

IDEAS ON HOW TO MEASURE PROGRESS

As previously mentioned, consistently meeting your macros goals leads to measurable progress in the following three areas:

- Physique: form, size, and development of your body
- Internal body functioning
- Relationship with food

Physical size, shape, and appearance are relevant and valid goals. But it's also important to have goals that go beyond the way we look and the number on the scale.

Appendix E: Ways to Measure Progress on page 189 offers a list of holistic ways to measure progress. Food is emotional and physical, and any change in your food behaviors offers an opportunity to learn more about yourself, your body's functioning, and your relationship with food.

ALL FOOD FITS

All foods fit in the macros method. A good metaphor to help conceptualize the macros framework is equating calories to money. Your daily calories are a daily budget, and macros targets are budget lines. You have a choice on how you spend your calories within each macros budget line every day.

With this said, most people find that they feel at their physical and mental/emotional best spending 80 to 90 percent of their daily calories on minimally processed whole foods like fruits, vegetables, high-quality proteins, nuts, seeds, and starches and whole grains.

The remaining 10 to 20 percent of the daily calorie budget can be spent on fun foods and treats, however you define them. There is nothing you cannot eat. You might think skipping the fun foods and treats is a "healthier" or faster way to reach your goals, but the opposite tends to be true. Banning any food with the intention of eliminating it usually intensifies the desire for it, triggering food cravings and overconsumption. On the other hand, eating a moderate amount of fun foods and treats every day is psychologically beneficial, as it provokes pleasure and increases self-trust around food. Eating a reasonably sized delicious dessert or a salty snack is not a crisis or mistake, it is just a pleasing moment every day. A useful rule of thumb is to enjoy one serving of a sweet or savory treat per day.

See Appendix F: Minimally Processed Whole Foods List on page 193.

LEARNING HOW TO EAT A
BALANCED MACROS MEAL

At the beginning of your macros journey, you will be making changes to your food and eating behaviours as you learn how to eat all foods in balance. Change can feel difficult and overwhelming sometimes, but the macros method is all about breaking meals down into building blocks: protein, carbohydrates, fat, micronutrients. This makes meal preparation a simple process of mix and match. Use my "Mix-and-Match Balanced Macros Plate" template on page 89 as a guide to help you:

- quickly put together meals without needing to follow a recipe;
- create an unlimited number of combinations for variety and pleasure;
- understand the correct portion sizes of each macronutrient that you require; and
- order balanced meals at restaurants and consume the right portion sizes for you.

It is especially helpful to use this meal template at the beginning to understand how easy it is to eat everything in balance and learn how to track individual foods and quantities to get specific calorie and macros breakdown at meals and snacks.

AFTER TRACKING: USE SIMPLE VISUAL GUIDELINES

We cannot and should not track indefinitely. So what happens after tracking for a period of time—either when you reach your goals or when you need to take a break? I was working with a nutrition expert and I wanted to stop tracking in detail, but I still wanted to have a system for eating in balance. They advised me to use two visual templates to help build a balanced meal with appropriate portion sizes.

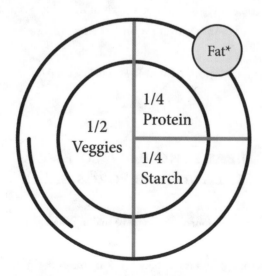

*Added fat quantities vary depending
on the fat content from the meat/protein.

The "Plate Method"[1]—a guide for dividing your plate into three proportional sections: mostly non-starchy vegetables, smaller amounts of starchy foods, and proteins.

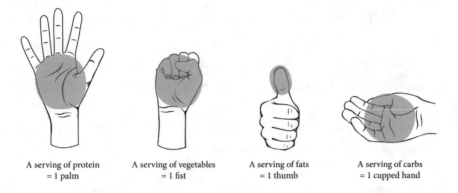

A serving of protein = 1 palm   A serving of vegetables = 1 fist   A serving of fats = 1 thumb   A serving of carbs = 1 cupped hand

"Hand-Size Portion Guide"[2]—using the palm of your hand and fingers as a reference for portion sizes for protein, carbohydrates and fats.

Both these methods are visual, simple, and portable. They help us to eat balanced meals and control portions and calories at every meal. If you are rolling your eyes about the use of the words "control" and "calories," I understand because these words are considered oppressive. At the same time, we are living in a historical moment where overconsumption of food is a primary health risk.

MACROS BALANCED EATING EVOLVES INTO AN EFFORTLESS HABIT

Ideally, we would all follow internal cues when making decisions about food. However, this assumes a body-mind precision where a person feels what macronutrient their body is hungry for and knows the right portion sizes to fuel it with.

---

[1] Aucoin, Nicole. Eating Your Favorite Foods with the Plate Method, 2021. Healthy Steps Nutrition. PDF download.

[2] St. Pierre, Brian. Portion Control Guide. Precision Nutrition. Infographic.

We might think that we have a "natural ability" to eat the right amount of food for our needs. But when it comes to food, our needs are more than just physical.

Most people's eating patterns have become disorganized by a combination of emotion and culture. We "eat our feelings" to cope with sadness *and* happiness. Food is omnipresent in our lives; ultra-processed foods are promoted, cheap, and readily available at the same time as we face social standards and pressures about weight loss and exercise. Eating based on emotion or cultural trends creates food-induced drama for the body and mind: calorie restriction, excessive calorie consumption, or following diets that advise totally eliminating, restricting, or overconsuming one macronutrient are all destabilizing.

Our internal hunger-satiety gauge may be hard to tune in to after years of ignoring it, manipulating food intake, and eating out of balance. All of this has diluted our "natural" hunger and satiety signals.

Eating a macros-balanced diet consistently, for a minimum of three months, is healing. It creates a habit of eating all the macronutrients and correct portion sizes. This habit creates a steady food routine that nourishes and therefore calms your body and mind. With time, our body-mind connection strengthens, laying the foundations for us to follow our internal bodily cues of hunger and satiety.

Consciously relearning what to eat and correct portion sizes ultimately makes eating in balance an effortless habit. In this way, we listen to and trust our bodies to inform our food choices, rather than allowing feelings or culture to drown out and override body-based intelligence.

MACROS AND DIET CULTURE

This book, and the macros method in general, is not meant to be used to abuse your body/mind. This approach to food is not meant to feed into an already toxic cultural context around body image, appearance, and food restriction. The goal of this way of eating is not to get as "skinny" as possible, because for most of us our lowest weight does not translate to physical health or emotional balance.

The pressure of social messaging about food and body image can manifest in seemingly opposite reactions, both of which are equally damaging to body, mind, and spirit:

- Overcompliance: forcing the body to survive on less food than it needs and exercising too much, in an attempt to meet unrealistic beauty standards and feel valued.
- Rejection: interpreting guidelines and recommendations for eating and movement as oppressive and controlling, and using overconsumption of food and neglect of the body as acts of rebellious empowerment.

Macros provides a moderate middle ground. When applied properly—as a tool that you use, rather than a system that you have to squeeze yourself into—the macros eating framework provides opportunities to:

- learn about how your body functions,
- improve your relationship with food,
- create lasting food behaviors that are essential for lifelong weight management, and
- experience peace of mind around the subject of food.

The more we can make food our ally and move away from an on-again, off-again approach, the better!

WORKING WITH A NUTRITION EXPERT

When using the macros framework to maintain, lose, or gain weight, it can be helpful to work with a nutritionist, dietician, or food coach for a period of time. When I decided to move forward from veganism to eat everything (kosher), I did not want a solitary, intellectual, psychologically intense experience with food and my body! I decided to work with a macros coach so I could learn from and lean on expert knowledge and guidance. It's a testament to how positive this experience was for me that I decided to write this book and share the knowledge I gained.

Hiring a nutrition expert to support you with food and eating choices and outcomes should be no different from hiring any other expert: it's a logical decision that saves time, simplifies the process, and reaps sustainable results.

A dietician, nutritionist, or food coach can help you:

- navigate complicated information and simplify decisions,
- create a personalized eating plan, and
- make food choices that actually lead to the results you want.

Specific to following a macros eating pattern, a dietician, nutritionist, and food coach helps to:

- set appropriate targets,
- calculate the number of calories you need to eat to reach your goals,
- calculate your macros percentages,
- clarify how long to be in a calorie deficit or surplus,
- teach you how to use the "plate method" and "hand portion size guide" to eat a balanced diet with correct portion sizes,
- guide you through the reverse dieting phase, and
- instruct you on how to maintain your weight after reaching a realistic weight goal for your height and age.

They can help you stop extreme approaches to eating and wellness, and spending hours and hours thinking and worrying about food.

For more about when to hire a nutrition expert and what qualifications to look for, see Appendix G: Working with a Nutrition Expert.

A NOTE ABOUT DIS-/ORDERED EATING

Food and eating always mean more to us than just the food we put into our mouths; what we eat (and desire to eat) is interwoven with our culture, personal history, emotions, and feelings.

If you have a history of disordered eating, this plan could be a therapeutic tool for you.

However, there is a delicate balance between mindfulness and obsession. If you notice that the macros method is causing you to obsess about food, your weight, and/or your body image and it is becoming all that you think about, it's a signal that you need to focus on improving your relationship with food.

Remain mindful that disordered eating sometimes manifests as excessively ordered eating, and seek support if you feel yourself becoming triggered by this eating framework.

WHEN FOOD AND MOVEMENT HABITS ARE NOT ENOUGH

Our society tells us that we should use willpower to change our appearance, thoughts, and feelings. By this reasoning, if we are unable to create change through our sheer willpower, then we are a failure and we need to keep trying harder.

However, there are legitimate cases when changing our food and movement behaviors is not enough to support our physical and mental/emotional health goals.

What we eat, how we move, health conditions, and hormones all have a huge influence on body size, thoughts, and feelings. If you feel that your best efforts are not resulting in the change you want, it does not mean you are a failure. There may be something else going on. Without delay or self-blame, you have the right to consult with nutrition experts and other specialists to explore medical and therapeutic interventions.

OPPORTUNITY TO MOVE OUR BODIES

Frequently, when we think of movement, we associate it with diet culture where exercise and movement are expressions of self-punishment for being "fat" or fear of becoming "fat." This toxic paradigm includes viewing eating as a reward for exercise or exercising to compensate for "overeating." That idea is not supportive and frankly misses the whole point of movement: your long-term comfort in your own body and mind!

Our ability to move our bodies regularly to support our physical and mental health is a tangible and accessible coping mechanism that we can rely on to manage physical and emotional stress and strain throughout our entire lives.

Moving our bodies:

- releases feel-good endorphins that help cope with pain, and dopamine that allows us to feel pleasure,
- allows us to take a break during our day, energize our bodies and refresh our minds,
- gives us time to process and regulate our emotions,
- strengthens the connection with the body we have, and
- boosts our mental capacity.

KOSHER FOOD LAWS, AT A GLANCE

The recipes in this book are organized into the three kosher food categories: meat, dairy, and pareve. The pareve foods are considered neutral and can be eaten with either milk or meat.

These three main principles inform a kosher diet:

1. Eat only fish that have fins and scales, and land animals that both chew the cud and have cleft hooves.

2. Meat and dairy are never mixed in recipes or served at the same meal.
3. Meat must be slaughtered in a kosher way, and drained of blood.

The laws of kosher are complex and extensive, and the above is a summary. For complete information, please talk to a rabbi or consult a book about kosher food laws.

ETHICAL CONSIDERATIONS FOR OMNIVORES

Being vegetarian and vegan for so many years made it difficult for me to transition to eating animal protein, even though my body was craving it. As I began to eat kosher meat and dairy products again, I realized that my choice was part of a modern moral dilemma. The practices underlying the production of meat and dairy are cruel and unsustainable: these include factory farming, slaughter methods that don't prioritize pain reduction, and feeding animals excessive antibiotics and hormones.

Working toward being an ethical omnivore means practicing restraint in some areas and taking action in others.

PRACTICE RESTRAINT

- Embrace the idea of correct portion size and quantities.
- Consume an adequate amount of animal products needed at various life stages.
- Release yourself from the habit of overcooking for family and guests and ordering too much food in restaurants.

TAKE ACTION

- Buy the most ethically produced animal products that your budget allows.

- Get familiar with a broad range of plant protein sources: tofu, tempeh, lentils, and beans, and include plant-based sources of protein in your daily and weekly dietary pattern.
- Minimize food waste in your home and while eating in restaurants.
- Use your consumer power to support sustainable animal husbandry practices rather than factory farming methods.
- Donate money and time to ethical food and animal welfare organizations.
- Share information about ethical animal consumption and meat reductionism to raise awareness.
- Ask about the origins of your food and its ingredients.
- Write to political representatives and religious leaders about the environmental impact of farming practices and food choices.

RECIPE SELECTION

All the recipes in this book are kosher, use everyday ingredients, and are simple to make.

Some of the recipes have a Jew-ish vibe, such as:

- Single-Serving Baked Shakshuka on page 19
- Lighter Potato Kugel on page 118
- Spinach and Ricotta Bourekas on page 129
- Marshmallow, Chocolate, and Graham Cracker Crembo Bites on page 147

Other recipes are modern food favorites that have been tweaked to balance the macros and meet kosher requirements. These include:

- Banana Blueberry Sheet Pan Protein Pancakes on page 5
- No Fuss Vegetarian Lasagna on page 94
- "Bacon" and Cheese Twice Baked Sweet Potatoes on page 105
- Oatmeal Chocolate Chip Cookies on page 151

The recipes in this book were developed to be mixed and matched in meal plans that give pleasure and meet daily macros goals. They are everyday recipes that you can cycle through, and some of them are special enough to serve for holiday meals and important occasions.

Each recipe provides nutritional information to make it easy for you to track your daily macros.

WHAT MATTERS MOST

There is no perfect body, and no person has perfect health. We cannot swap our body for someone else's. We can only accept the body we have and give it the care it needs to be able to carry us through life.

We can remember the instruction in the Hebrew Bible/Tanakh: "Shmor Nafshecha: Guard Your Health." This verse in Deuteronomy 4:15 obligates us to take actions to guard our own life and prevent damage to our body.

The ways we can guard our own life include: eating in balance; following safety laws and hygiene best practices; maintaining healthy physical and mental/emotional routines such as getting proper rest and sleep; moving our bodies regularly; developing a positive attitude; and participating in supportive and loving relationships. When we are in good physical and mental health, it places us in a better position to do good in our families and communities.

The goal of the macros eating plan is balance and moderation: not too much, not too little, nothing is banned. You can experience peace with food, be at ease in your body, and have the energy to do what you feel called to do in this life with joy.

When I started using this method in June 2021, my goals were to:

- relearn how to eat a balanced diet of all (kosher) food,

- reach and maintain a reasonable body weight,
- feel emotionally balanced,
- have the energy to move my body every day in the way that I enjoy, and
- reconnect with the pleasure of eating and sharing meals with others.

I feel that the macros framework has helped me do all of this and more. One change I am particularly grateful for is that the macros framework has allowed me to create a more balanced and joyful food environment with my husband and daughter.

I hope that the macros method and these recipes support your best intentions for achieving physical health and emotional balance.

I am so glad that you are here.

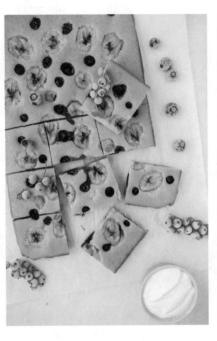
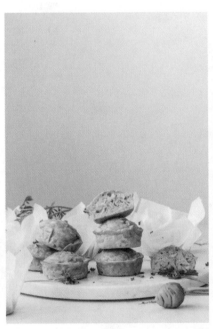
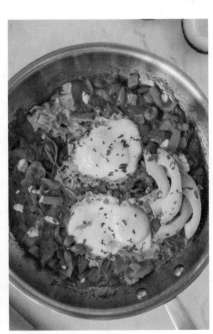

BREAKFAST RECIPES

BAKED SALMON CAKES

PAREVE

Prep time: 20 minutes | Cook time: 20 minutes | Total time: 40 minutes

Yield: 5 cakes

This baked salmon cake is perfect for an open-faced breakfast bagel sandwich. It is made with canned salmon and tuna fish, so it is super easy to have the ingredients on hand. The version here uses a combination of fish, which you could adapt according to taste and what's in your pantry. A delicious everyday twist on the classic smoked salmon cream cheese bagel, these fish cakes can also be served for lunch or dinner.

Ingredients

- 8 ounces (230g) canned salmon, water-packed
- 4 ounces (115g) canned tuna, water-packed
- 2 eggs, beaten
- 1 tablespoon ground flaxseed
- ½ cup (45g) rolled oats
- 3 scallions, white and light green parts only
- 1 teaspoon garlic powder
- Salt and pepper to taste

Variations
- Add fresh parsley or basil to the fish mix before baking for more flavor.

- Replace rolled oats with bread crumbs to change the texture a little bit.
- For Passover, use quinoa flakes instead of rolled oats.

Tools

- Can opener
- Kitchen scale
- Measuring cups and spoons
- Medium mixing bowl
- Parchment paper
- Rimmed baking sheet
- Spatula

Instructions

1. Preheat the oven to 350°F (180°C).

2. Line a baking sheet with oiled parchment paper.

3. Drain the salmon and tuna and place them into a medium mixing bowl.

4. Add the eggs, flaxseed, oats, scallions, and garlic powder. Season with salt and pepper and mix well. Let the mixture sit for 10 minutes so the oats can absorb the egg liquid.

5. After resting, if the mixture still seems too wet, add a couple more tablespoons of oats until the mixture has a consistency that will hold its shape in patties.

6. Use your hands to shape the fish mixture into five even patties, and place them on the prepared baking sheet.

7. Cook for 20 minutes, flipping halfway through. The cakes are done when they're crispy on both sides.

8. Serve hot or cold.

Serving Suggestions

- Serve on half of a whole-wheat bagel or with some whole-grain bread.

- Serve with cream cheese, tomato, cucumber, and red onion.

- Serve as a lunch or dinner option on top of a green salad.

Serving size: 1 salmon cake
Calories per serving: 142
Macros: Carbohydrates: 6.5g; Fiber: 1g; Protein: 16g; Fat: 6g

BANANA BLUEBERRY SHEET PAN PROTEIN PANCAKES

PAREVE

Prep time: 10 minutes | Cook time: 20 minutes | Total time: 30 minutes

Yield: 16 squares

These gluten- and dairy-free sheet pan protein pancakes come together in less than ten minutes and taste like individual pancakes without all the work! Topped with Greek yogurt and fresh fruit, this is a special sweet and soft cake-like breakfast. This recipe is easy to make in advance and warm up or take on the go.

Ingredients

- 2 eggs
- 2 egg whites (¼ cup)
- 1 cup (240ml) unsweetened soy milk
- 2 tablespoons maple syrup (or honey)
- 2 teaspoons apple cider vinegar
- 1 teaspoon vanilla extract
- 2 cups (240g) fine almond flour
- ½ teaspoon baking soda
- ½ teaspoon baking powder
- ¼ teaspoon salt

- 2 bananas, sliced
- 1 cup (150g) fresh or frozen blueberries

Optional Garnish

- ¼ cup Greek yogurt on each pancake square
- Extra blueberries, for serving

Variations

- Switch out the blueberries for any fresh or frozen berries of your choice.
- Use chocolate chips and a peanut butter swirl for a different flavor.

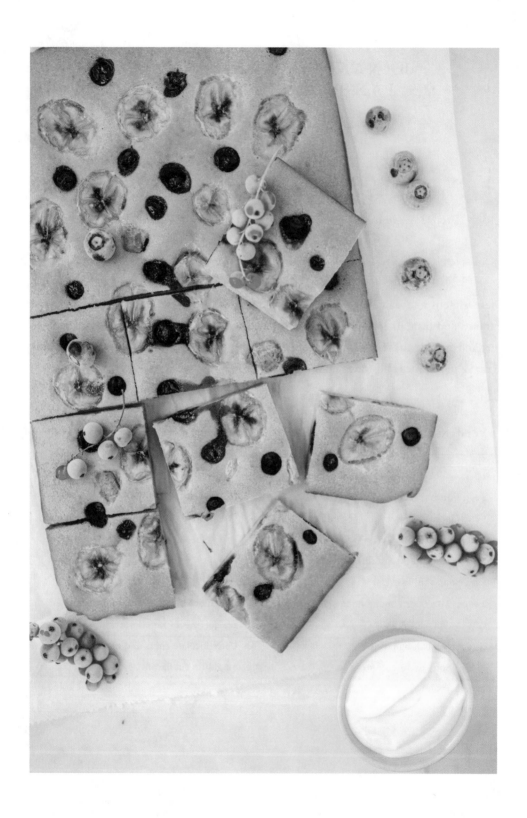

Tools

- Cutting board
- Kitchen scale
- Large mixing bowl
- Measuring cups and spoons
- Parchment paper
- Rimmed baking sheet (18 x 13-inch/45 x 33 cm)
- Sharp knife
- Spatula
- Whisk

Instructions

1. Preheat the oven to 350°F (180°C) and line a rimmed baking sheet with a piece of parchment paper.
2. In a large mixing bowl, combine eggs, egg whites, soy milk, maple syrup, vinegar, and vanilla. Whisk until smooth and slightly fluffy.
3. Add in the almond flour, baking soda, baking powder, and salt. Gently fold the dry ingredients into the wet until everything is combined and smooth.
4. Pour the batter onto the prepared baking sheet and top with sliced bananas and blueberries.
5. Transfer to the oven to bake until golden brown and puffed up, around 18 to 20 minutes. Remove from the oven and set aside to cool for at least 15 minutes.
6. Slice into 16 pancake squares and top each portion with ¼ cup of Greek yogurt and a handful of fresh blueberries.

WITHOUT YOGURT
Serving size: 1 pancake square
Calories per serving: 116
Macros: Carbohydrates: 9.6g; Fiber: 3g; Protein: 4.5g; Fat: 6.6g

WITH YOGURT
Serving size: 1 pancake square, with yogurt
Calories per serving: 120
Macros: Carbohydrates: 10.1g; Fiber: 3g; Protein: 4.6g; Fat: 6.7g

BERRY PROTEIN SMOOTHIE BOWL

PAREVE

Prep time: 5 minutes

Yield: 1 serving

This sweet and filling berry protein smoothie bowl comes together in less than five minutes and is packed with protein and fiber. Unlike a traditional smoothie, this smoothie has a thick consistency and you can eat it in a bowl with a spoon, which feels more satisfying. The recipe calls for vegan protein powder. It's best to use a whole food source that is under 150 calories and has at least 20 grams of protein per serving.

Ingredients

- 1 cup (150g) mixed frozen berries
- ½ frozen banana
- 1 scoop vegan protein powder, any flavor with 20 grams protein per serving
- ¼ cup (60ml) unsweetened soy milk
- 1 cup (30g) baby spinach
- 1 teaspoon unsweetened peanut butter
- ½ teaspoon vanilla extract

Variations

- Use just one type of frozen berry for a simpler flavor.
- Use frozen pineapple and coconut milk for a decadent tropical twist.
- Replace the peanut butter with almond, tahini, or sunflower seed butter.

Tools

- Blender or food processor
- Kitchen scale
- Measuring cups and spoons
- Serving bowl

Instructions

1. Place the berries, banana, protein powder, soy milk, spinach, peanut butter, and vanilla into a high-speed blender or food processor and blend until completely smooth and creamy.
2. Transfer to a serving bowl and decorate with preferred toppings from the serving options list.
3. Serve while still cold and thick.

Serving Options

- Add chopped or whole almonds, cashews, walnuts, or pumpkin seeds.
- Garnish with shredded coconut, chia seeds, or hemp hearts.

Serving size: 1 smoothie bowl
Calories per serving (toppings not included): 290
Macros: Carbohydrates: 40g; Fiber: 8g; Protein: 28g; Fat: 4g

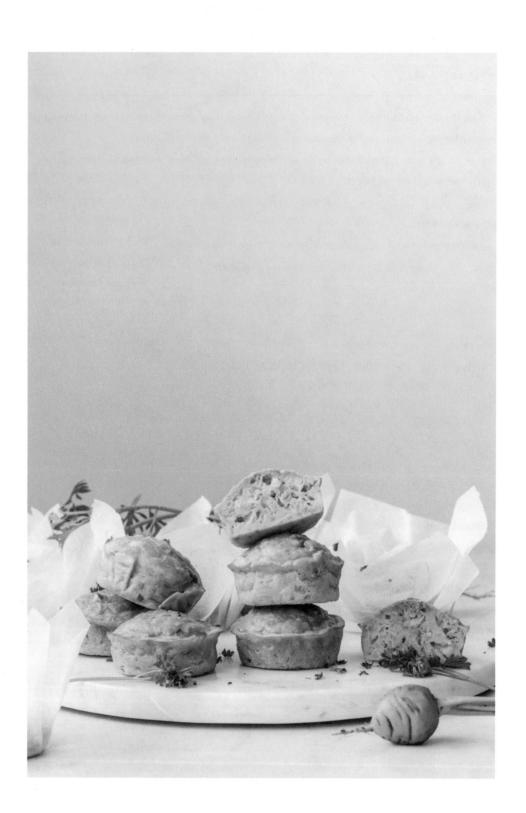

BOKER TOV PROTEIN MUFFINS

Prep time: 10 minutes | Cook time: 20 minutes | Total time: 30 minutes

Yield: 12 muffins

These morning apple, carrot, zucchini, and cranberry muffins are moist and perfectly spiced. You can bake the whole batch on the weekend, or even double the recipe and enjoy them as a portable breakfast or snack all week long.

Ingredients

- 1 medium zucchini, shredded
- 2 medium carrots, shredded
- 1 medium apple, shredded
- 3 large eggs
- ½ cup (140g) Greek yogurt
- 3 tablespoons coconut oil, melted
- ¼ cup (60ml) pure maple syrup
- 1 teaspoon pure vanilla extract
- 2 cups (250g) whole-wheat flour
- 1 teaspoon baking soda
- 1½ teaspoons baking powder
- 1 teaspoon cinnamon
- ½ teaspoon ground ginger
- ½ cup (35g) almonds, chopped
- ½ cup (65g) unsweetened dried cranberries

Variations

- Replace the whole-wheat flour with all-purpose gluten-free flour.
- Swap the cranberries for raisins or diced dried apricots.
- Replace the almonds with walnuts, pecans, pumpkin seeds, etc.

Tools

- Cooking oil spray
- Grater
- Kitchen scale
- Large mixing bowl
- Measuring cups and spoons
- Muffin tin
- Paper muffin liners (optional)
- Rubber spatula
- Small mixing bowl
- Vegetable peeler
- Whisk

Instructions

1. Preheat the oven to 360°F (180°C) and line a 12-cup muffin tin with paper liners. Alternatively, you can spray the muffin tin with nonstick baking spray.
2. In a large mixing bowl, combine zucchini, carrots, apple, eggs, Greek yogurt, coconut oil, maple syrup, and vanilla. Whisk until combined.
3. In a separate smaller bowl, combine the flour, baking soda, baking powder, cinnamon, and ginger.
4. Add the dry ingredients into the wet and gently fold together until everything is just combined. Don't overmix.
5. Fold in the almonds and dried cranberries.
6. Divide the batter between the 12 muffin cups and place in the preheated oven. Bake until the muffins are deep golden brown in color and a toothpick inserted into the center comes out clean or with a few moist crumbs, around 18 to 20 minutes.
7. Leave to cool for at least 20 minutes before removing from the muffin tin.

Serving size: 1 muffin (about 100 grams per muffin)
Calories per serving: 167
Macros: Carbohydrates: 29g; Fiber: 4g; Protein: 5.4g; Fat: 4.1g

COTTAGE CHEESE AND FRUIT
BREAKFAST PARFAIT

Prep time: 5 minutes

Yield: 1 serving

A quick and simple fruit and cottage cheese breakfast parfait. You just throw everything together in a bowl and eat immediately, or pack it into a jar for a portable breakfast. This balanced meal has protein from the cottage cheese, healthy fat from the nuts, and fiber and micronutrients from the fruit.

Ingredients

- ¾ cup (170g) low-fat cottage cheese
- ¼ cup (70g) low-fat Greek yogurt
- 1 teaspoon honey or maple syrup
- ½ teaspoon vanilla extract
- ½ banana, sliced
- ¼ cup (50g) fresh pineapple, diced
- 1 kiwi, sliced
- 1 teaspoon chia seeds
- 1 teaspoon unsweetened coconut flakes

Variations

- Use berries and peanut butter for a PB&J variation.
- Add sliced avocado, cherry tomatoes, chopped cucumber, and a cooked egg to turn it into a savory breakfast parfait.
- Add muesli, rolled oats, or quinoa flakes if you want a higher carbohydrate breakfast.

Tools

- Cutting board
- Kitchen scale
- Measuring cups and spoons
- Serving bowl or a glass jar
- Sharp knife
- Spoon

Instructions

1. Add cottage cheese, Greek yogurt, honey, and vanilla to a bowl or glass jar and briefly stir.

2. Top with banana, pineapple, kiwi, chia seeds, and coconut flakes.

3. Serve immediately or pack in a jar as a portable meal.

Serving size: 1 cottage cheese parfait
Calories per serving: 330
Macros: Carbohydrates: 44g; Fiber: 5g; Protein: 32g; Fat: 6g

CREAMY ZUCCHINI PROTEIN OVERNIGHT OATS

DAIRY

Prep time: 10 minutes

Yield: 2 servings

These creamy and delicious zucchini protein overnight oats are made the night before and work as a great on-the-go breakfast that you can take to work or school. Zucchini is not often on the morning menu, but its mild flavor makes it a great choice for adding micronutrients and fiber to breakfast. The oats swell up to become sweet and pudding-like after overnight soaking.

Ingredients

- ½ cup (45g) rolled oats
- ½ cup (120ml) low-fat milk
- ½ cup (140g) low-fat plain Greek yogurt
- 1 scoop vanilla protein powder
- ½ cup (60g) shredded zucchini
- 1 teaspoon honey or maple syrup
- ½ teaspoon vanilla extract
- 1 tablespoon unsweetened peanut butter
- 1 cup (100g) fresh or frozen strawberries, chopped

Variations

- Use blueberries and almond butter for a different flavor combination.
- Use sliced mango or passion fruit for a tropical twist.
- Use unsweetened soy milk and coconut yogurt for a vegan option.

Tools

- Glass jar with lid
- Grater
- Kitchen scale
- Measuring cups and spoons
- Spoon

Instructions

1. Place oats, milk, Greek yogurt, protein powder, zucchini, honey, and vanilla in a glass jar and stir to combine.
2. Top with peanut butter and strawberries.
3. Screw on the lid and place in the fridge overnight.

Serving size: 1 serving (½ jar of overnight oats)
Calories per serving: 304
Macros: Carbohydrates: 32g; Fiber: 5g; Protein: 25g; Fat: 10g

OAT, PUMPKIN, AND ALMOND BUTTER BREAKFAST BARS

PAREVE

Prep time: 10 minutes | Cook time: 20 minutes | Total time: 30 minutes

Yield: 6 or 8 bars

Moist and tender, these bars come together in less than thirty minutes and work as a great breakfast-on-the-go option. You can double the batch and your whole family will enjoy them all week long for breakfast or a snack. They are high in fiber, protein, and nutrients.

Ingredients

- 2 cups (180g) rolled oats
- ½ cup (110g) pumpkin puree
- ½ cup (120g) natural almond butter
- 1 cup (220g) egg whites
- ¼ cup (60ml) honey or maple syrup
- 2 teaspoons pumpkin pie spice
- 1 teaspoon pure vanilla extract
- ½ cup (60g) pumpkin seeds

Variations
- Replace the pumpkin with mashed banana for a banana bread bar version.
- Use peanut butter instead of almond butter.
- Use quinoa or millet flakes instead of rolled oats for a gluten-free option.

- Toss in different add-ins to make them slightly different every single time: dried cranberries, chopped dried apricots, walnuts, slivered almonds.

Tools

- Cutting board
- Kitchen scale
- Large mixing bowl
- Measuring cups and spoons
- Parchment paper
- Rimmed baking sheet (18 x 13-inch / 45 x 33 cm)
- Rubber spatula
- Sharp knife

Instructions

1. Preheat the oven to 375°F (190°C) and line a rimmed baking sheet with a piece of parchment paper.
2. In a large mixing bowl, combine rolled oats, pumpkin puree, almond butter, egg whites, honey, pumpkin pie spice, and vanilla. Mix until everything is incorporated.
3. Transfer the mixture to the prepared baking sheet and top with pumpkin seeds.
4. Place in the oven to bake until the bars are golden and set, around 20 to 25 minutes.
5. Remove from the oven and allow to cool for 20 minutes before slicing.

Serving size: 1 bar

IF MAKING 6 BARS
Calories per serving: 400
Macros: Carbohydrates: 39.5g; Fiber: 7g; Protein: 25g; Fat: 22g

IF MAKING 8 BARS
Calories per serving: 300
Macros: Carbohydrates: 29.5g; Fiber: 5g; Protein: 18g; Fat: 16.4g

SINGLE-SERVING BAKED SHAKSHUKA

DAIRY

Prep time: 5 minutes | Cook time: 20 minutes | Total time: 25 minutes

Yield: 1 serving

Perfectly baked eggs in a rich, spiced tomato sauce with a dollop of creamy cottage cheese and some fresh herbs to brighten everything up. This flavorsome dish works well for any meal of the day, and the fact that it is single serve gives built-in portion control.

Ingredients

- 1 teaspoon olive oil
- 1 scallion, thinly sliced
- ½ red bell pepper, chopped
- 2 small tomatoes, chopped
- 1 garlic clove, minced
- ½ teaspoon ground cumin
- ¼ teaspoon smoked paprika
- 1 medium egg
- 2 egg whites (¼ cup)
- 1 ounce (28g) halloumi cheese, crumbled
- ¼ cup (15g) fresh parsley, chopped
- Salt and pepper to taste

Variations

- Use a green pepper instead of the red one, and add some spinach and kale to the sauce for a green twist on the classic shakshuka.
- Skip the eggs and use crumbled tofu for a vegan option.
- Add another egg to boost richness and protein.
- Add some harissa paste to the sauce to add spicy heat.
- Serve alongside avocado.

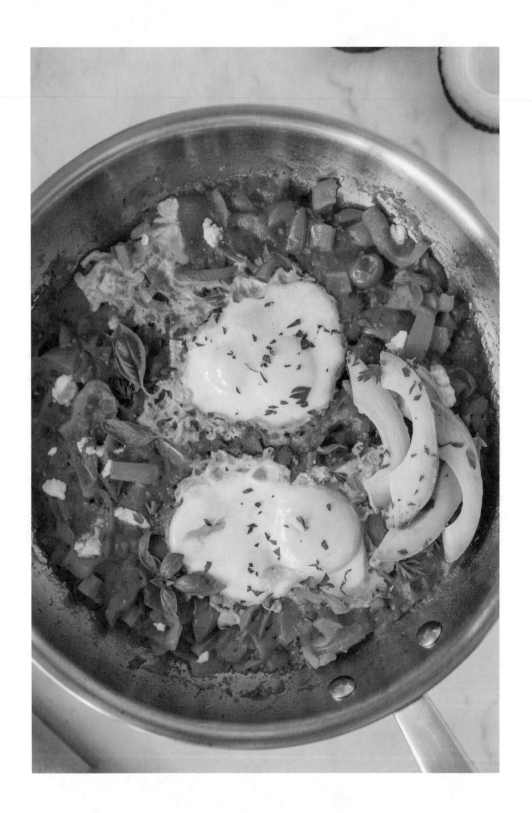

Tools

- Cooking oil spray
- Cutting board
- Kitchen scale
- Measuring cups and spoons
- Sharp knife
- Skillet
- Small oven-proof dish
- Spatula

Instructions

1. Preheat the oven to 350°F (180°C) and spray a small baking dish with some nonstick baking spray.
2. Heat olive oil in a skillet over medium heat.
3. Add scallion, red bell pepper, and tomatoes; season with salt and pepper to taste. Cook, stirring occasionally, until the vegetables are soft, around 6 to 7 minutes.
4. Add the garlic, cumin, and smoked paprika; continue cooking for another 1 to 2 minutes.
5. Transfer the tomato mixture to the prepared baking dish. Crack in the egg and add 2 egg whites. Season the eggs with salt and pepper to taste.
6. Place the baking dish into the oven and bake until the eggs are done to your liking—around 6 minutes for very runny yolks or 10 minutes for firmer eggs.
7. Remove the baking dish from the oven and top with halloumi and fresh parsley.

Serving size: 1 shakshuka
Calories per serving: 312
Macros: Carbohydrates: 19g; Fiber: 5g; Protein: 25g; Fat: 17g

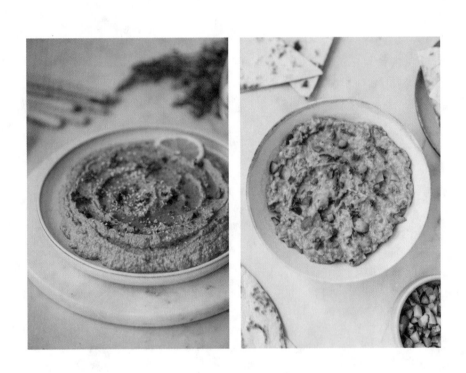

DIPS AND SPREADS

BEET AND RICOTTA DIP

Prep time: 10 minutes | Cook time: 40 minutes | Total time: 50 minutes

Yield: 4 servings

A rich and earthy dip made from baked beets and ricotta cheese, with a vibrant pink color. This dip has a nice citrus tang from sumac, a spice from a fruit berry that grows and is commonly used in cooking in the Middle East.

Ingredients

- 4 medium beets
- 1 cup (250g) ricotta cheese
- Juice of 1 lemon
- 1 teaspoon sumac (optional)
- Salt and pepper to taste
- 2 tablespoons fresh mint, thinly sliced, for garnish

Variations
- Use Greek yogurt or cottage cheese instead of ricotta.
- Top the dip with some toasted walnuts or pine nuts for crunch.
- Swap out the beets for pumpkin for a flavor and color variation.

Tools

- Aluminum foil
- Cutting board
- Food processor
- Kitchen scale
- Measuring cups and spoons
- Rimmed baking sheet
- Sharp knife

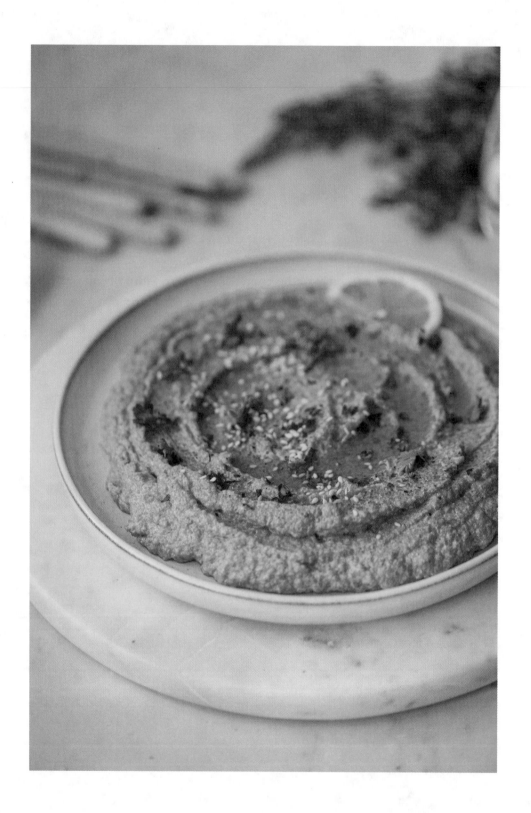

Instructions

1. Preheat the oven to 400°F (200°C).

2. Wrap each beet in a piece of aluminum foil and place it on a rimmed baking sheet. Transfer to the oven and roast until the beets are tender when pierced with a knife, around 35 to 40 minutes.

3. Allow beets to cool slightly and peel under running water.

4. Transfer beets to the bowl of a food processor and add the ricotta, lemon juice, sumac, and a large pinch of salt and pepper. Process until a smooth and creamy dip forms. If needed, you can add a splash of water to adjust the consistency.

5. Taste and adjust the seasoning and place the dip into a serving dish. Garnish with fresh mint and serve.

Serving size: ¼ recipe
Calories per serving: 125
Macros: Carbohydrates: 11.8g; Fiber: 2g; Protein: 8.5g; Fat: 5.2g

EGG AND ONION SPREAD

PAREVE

Prep time: 10 minutes | Cooking time: 10 minutes | Total time: 20 minutes

Yield: 4 servings

This simple egg and onion spread recipe offers a few minor updates to a classic and enduring recipe. The recipe calls for fewer egg yolks and uses walnut oil instead of schmaltz. This recipe feels and tastes like "spring on a plate" with eggs and green onions. It's delicious served with matzo, rice cakes, or bread.

Ingredients

- 6 large eggs
- 1 medium red onion
- 1 green onion (scallion), chopped
- 1 teaspoon Dijon mustard
- 1 teaspoon lemon juice
- 1 teaspoon walnut oil
- ½ teaspoon smoked paprika
- Salt and pepper to taste

Tools

- Cutting board
- Kitchen scale
- Measuring cups and spoons
- Mixing bowl
- Sharp knife
- Small saucepan with lid
- Spoon

Instructions

1. Place the eggs in a small pot and cover with water. Place over high heat, cover, and bring to a boil. Once boiling, turn off the heat and leave the pot to stand with the lid still on. The eggs should be perfectly hard-boiled after sitting for 10 to 12 minutes.

2. Meanwhile, peel and finely chop the red onion and transfer it to a mixing bowl.

3. Rinse the eggs under cold water, and peel them.

4. Remove the yolks from 3 of the eggs and set them aside for another use.

5. Finely chop the remaining 3 egg whites and 3 whole eggs, and transfer to the mixing bowl with red onion.

6. Add chopped scallion and Dijon mustard, drizzle with lemon juice and walnut oil, and season with smoked paprika, salt, and pepper. Gently mix to combine.

7. Taste and add more salt and pepper if desired.

Serving size: ¼ recipe
Calories per serving: 108
Macros: Carbohydrates: 5g; Fiber: 1g; Protein: 10g; Fat: 5g

LEMONY WHITE BEAN DIP WITH GARLIC AND ZAATAR

Prep time: 10 minutes

Yield: 4 servings

This lemony white bean dip with garlic and zaatar hits all the right notes with the creaminess from the white beans, the zesty freshness from the lemons, and the nutty herbal kick from the zaatar and garlic. This recipe works both as a dip and as a sandwich spread.

Ingredients

- 1 14-ounce can (390g) white beans, rinsed and drained (or cooked from scratch)
- 1 tablespoon extra-virgin olive oil
- Juice of 1 lemon (or more depending on how lemony you like it)
- 1 garlic clove
- 1 to 2 tablespoons zaatar
- Salt and pepper to taste

Variations

- Use chickpeas or fava beans for a flavor variation.
- Add roasted red peppers or eggplant to the dip for extra vegetable, color, and moisture.
- Serve with fresh sliced crunchy vegetables, crackers, or pita bread for dipping.
- Replace zaatar with dried thyme, sesame seeds, and lemon zest.

Tools

- Citrus juicer
- Colander
- Cutting board
- Food processor
- Kitchen scale
- Measuring cups and spoons
- Sharp knife

Instructions

1. Add the drained white beans to a food processor and process for a couple of seconds to mash.

2. Add in the olive oil, lemon juice, garlic, and zaatar. Season with a pinch of salt and pepper and process until smooth and creamy.

3. If it seems too thick, add 1 to 2 tablespoons of water at a time, until you reach your desired consistency. Taste and adjust the seasoning with more salt, pepper, or zaatar.

4. Transfer to a serving plate and sprinkle extra zaatar on top before serving.

Serving size: ¼ recipe

Calories per serving: 167

Macros: Carbohydrates: 24.6g; Fiber: 5g; Protein: 8.5g; Fat: 4.4g

PICKLED HERRING WITH ONION, SOUR CREAM, AND A LITTLE RASPBERRY JAM

Prep time: 10 minutes

Yield: 6 servings

I grew up with this recipe as my grandmother always served herring, onions, and sour cream dip with crackers. It can also be enjoyed as a healthy snack, in place of meat for a meal, or served at a kiddush. The marinated herring is salty, the sour cream is silky, and the raspberry jam adds a pop of sweetness! This is delicious served on toasted rye bread.

Ingredients

- 12 ounces (340g) jarred herring in wine sauce
- ½ onion, sliced thin
- ½ cup (100g) low-fat sour cream
- 1 teaspoon brown sugar
- 2 teaspoons wine sauce brine (reserved from the jarred herring)
- 1 tablespoon raspberry jam (optional)
- Chopped parsley for garnish

Variations

- Add ¼ cup chopped dried cranberries to increase color, texture, and tartness.
- For a more traditional recipe, skip the raspberry jam.

Tools

- Colander
- Cutting board
- Kitchen scale
- Measuring cups and spoons
- Medium mixing bowl
- Rubber spatula
- Sharp knife
- Small mixing bowl
- Spoon

Instructions

1. Drain herring in a colander, reserving 2 tablespoons of the wine sauce for later. Discard the onions from the jar.
2. Cut the herring into bite-size pieces.
3. Place thinly sliced onion in a medium mixing bowl.
4. Add the herring to the bowl with the onions, and fold in the sour cream.
5. Add brown sugar, wine brine, and jam.
6. Refrigerate for at least one hour before serving.
7. Place the dip into a small serving bowl and garnish with chopped parsley.

Serving size: 1/6 recipe

WITHOUT RASPBERRY JAM
Calories per serving: 106
Macros: Carbohydrates: 14.3g; Fiber: 0g; Protein: 7.4g; Fat: 2g

WITH RASPBERRY JAM
Calories per serving: 115
Macros: Carbohydrates: 16.5g; Fiber: 0g; Protein: 7.5g; Fat: 2g

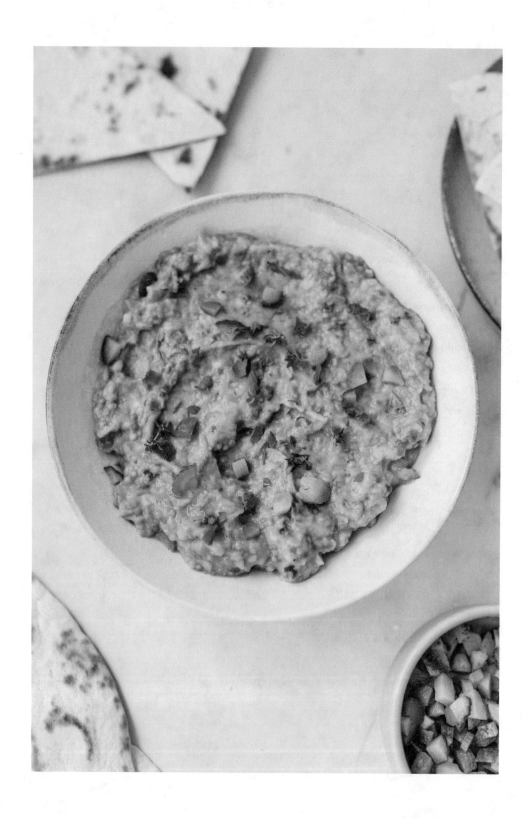

ROASTED EGGPLANT AND PICKLE DIP

PAREVE

Prep time: 10 minutes | Cook time: 45 minutes | Total time: 55 minutes

Yield: 4 servings

This dip is a play on the traditional baba ganoush. Eggplant and pickles create a unique flavor combination that combines the best of both worlds: rich and creamy with crunchy and tangy. This dip also works as a spread for pita bread with hummus or roasted meat with fresh vegetables.

Ingredients

- 2 medium eggplants, washed and dried
- 2 garlic cloves, minced
- Juice of 1 lemon
- 3 tablespoons tahini
- ¼ teaspoon ground coriander
- ½ teaspoon ground cumin
- ½ cup (71g) diced pickles
- ½ cup (30g) fresh parsley, chopped
- Salt and pepper to taste

Variations

- Replace the eggplant with roasted zucchini for a flavor variation.
- Skip the tahini and use Greek yogurt or cottage cheese for extra protein.

Tools

- Citrus juicer
- Cutting board
- Fork
- Kitchen scale
- Measuring cups and spoons
- Medium mixing bowl
- Parchment paper
- Rimmed baking sheet
- Sharp knife

Instructions

1. Preheat the oven to 400°F (200°C) and line a rimmed baking sheet with a piece of parchment paper.

2. Pierce the eggplants a couple of times with a fork and place on the prepared baking sheet. Transfer to the oven to roast until completely tender, around 35 to 40 minutes.

3. Remove from the oven and set aside to cool for 10 minutes.

4. Once the eggplants are cool enough to handle, peel them and transfer the flesh to a mixing bowl. Mash the eggplant flesh with a fork.

5. Add the garlic, lemon juice, tahini, coriander, cumin, pickles, and parsley; season with a pinch of salt and pepper. Mix well, taste, and adjust the seasoning with more salt, pepper, cumin, or coriander, if needed.

6. Transfer to a serving plate and garnish with a few extra pickle slices and fresh parsley.

Serving size: ¼ recipe
Calories per serving: 137
Macros: Carbohydrates: 18.6g; Fiber: 9g; Protein: 4.7g; Fat: 6.6g

ROASTED GARLIC, YOGURT, TURMERIC, AND MINT DIP

DAIRY

Prep time: 10 minutes | Cook time: 45 minutes | Total time: 55 minutes

Yield: 6 servings

This tasty creamy dip is perfect to serve with freshly cut vegetables, crackers, or with challah for Shabbat.

Ingredients

- Roasted head of garlic, use an amount to taste
- 1 teaspoon olive oil
- 2 or more chive scapes, chopped
- 5 mint leaves, chopped
- ½ teaspoon salt
- ½ teaspoon apple cider vinegar
- ½ teaspoon coconut brown sugar
- ½ teaspoon turmeric
- Black pepper, to taste
- 1½ cups (425g) full-fat plain Greek yogurt, divided

Variations

- Make yogurt sauce by putting all the ingredients in the blender until smooth. This sauce goes especially well with breakfast salmon cakes, baked salmon, or as a dressing for a pareve salad.
- If you are short on time, use just one clove of raw garlic instead of the roasted garlic.

Tools

- Aluminum foil
- Colander
- Cutting board
- Food processor or blender
- Kitchen scale
- Measuring cups and spoons
- Rimmed baking sheet
- Sharp knife
- Small serving bowl
- Spoon

Instructions

1. Heat the oven to 400°F (200°C).
2. Peel the outer layers of skin from the garlic head and cut off the top. Rub it with olive oil, wrap in aluminum foil, and place on a baking sheet.
3. Transfer to the oven and bake for 40 to 45 minutes, until the cloves are soft and golden brown in color.
4. Place the garlic, chives, mint, salt, vinegar, brown sugar, turmeric, and black pepper in a food processor or small blender.
5. Add ¼ cup yogurt and pulse until just blended, to a thick paste.
6. Gently stir the spiced garlic yogurt into 1¼ cup yogurt in a bowl. Note: if you do this step in the blender, the consistency will be that of a runny sauce rather than a thick dip.
7. Add more garlic, salt, pepper, chopped chives, and mint to taste.
8. Serve with crackers or raw cut vegetables.

Serving size: ⅙ recipe
Calories per serving: 66
Macros: Carbohydrates: 3.5g; Fiber: 1g; Protein: 5.2g; Fat: 3.5g

TUNA FISH SPREAD

DAIRY

Prep time: 5 minutes

Yield: 1 serving

One of the foods I craved most during my vegan years was tuna fish. The recipe below uses low-fat Greek yogurt and a touch of mayonnaise to create a creamy tuna spread to serve as a dip, sandwich filling, or to add to a salad.

Ingredients

- 1 (5-ounce / 113g) can tuna packed in water, drained
- ¼ cup (56g) low-fat Greek yogurt
- 1 teaspoon mayonnaise
- 1 tablespoon fresh lemon juice or white vinegar
- 1 celery stalk, finely chopped
- ¼ red or yellow onion, diced small
- Salt and freshly ground black pepper

Tools

- Citrus juicer
- Cutting board
- Kitchen scale
- Measuring cups and spoons
- Sharp knife
- Small mixing bowl x 2
- Spoon

Variations

- Replace the canned tuna with canned salmon.
- Add diced pickles or capers.
- Use cottage cheese instead of yogurt.
- Serve on toast and melt a slice of cheese on top for a lovely tuna melt. Cheeses like Cheddar, Swiss, Havarti, and mozzarella all work.

Instructions

1. Place drained tuna fish in a bowl and use your hands to break it into smaller pieces.
2. In another bowl, mix together the Greek yogurt, mayonnaise, and lemon juice until well combined into a dressing.
3. Add the chopped celery and red onion to the tuna.
4. Pour the dressing over the tuna mix and stir until well combined. Add salt and pepper to taste.

Serving size: 1 serving

Calories per serving: 247

Macros: Carbohydrates: 12g; Fiber: 2g; Protein: 32g; Fat: 7g

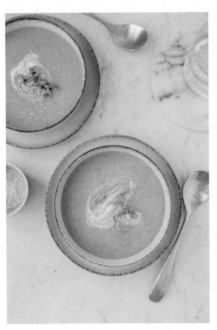
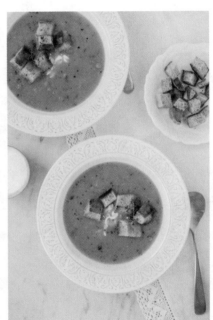

SOUPS

RED LENTIL, TOMATO, AND COCONUT SOUP

PAREVE

Prep time: 10 minutes | Cook time: 20 to 25 minutes | Total time: 35 minutes

Yield: 6 servings

This spiced lentil soup recipe is trouble free and delicious with a creamy, rich undertone from the tomatoes and coconut milk. Red lentils have a slightly sweet and nutty taste, which combines with the tomatoes and spices to create a flavorful, satisfying soup.

Ingredients

- 1 teaspoon coconut oil
- 2 tablespoons water
- 1 medium red onion, finely chopped
- 2 shallots, finely chopped
- 1 garlic clove, minced
- 1 cup (200g) dried red lentils
- 1 (14.5-ounce / 400g) can crushed tomatoes
- ¾ cup (175ml) unsweetened light coconut milk, shaken well
- 2 teaspoons cumin
- 1 teaspoon coriander
- ½ teaspoon turmeric powder
- ⅛ teaspoon cinnamon
- Add ⅛ teaspoon cayenne pepper for heat
- 4 cups (945ml) vegetable stock
- Salt and freshly ground pepper to taste

Tools

- Cutting board
- Immersion blender
- Kitchen scale
- Measuring cups and spoons
- Sharp knife
- Spatula
- Stock pot (4 liter)
- Vegetable peeler

Instructions

---

1. To a stock pot set over medium heat, add the coconut oil and water.

2. Add the onions and shallots and sauté until the onions are translucent, about 5 minutes. Add the garlic and continue to cook for 2 minutes.

3. Add the lentils, tomatoes, coconut milk, cumin, coriander, turmeric, cinnamon, and cayenne pepper and mix evenly.

4. Add vegetable stock and bring to a boil, then simmer uncovered for 20 to 25 minutes until the lentils are soft but not mushy.

5. Add salt and pepper to taste.

6. Serve hot.

Serving size: ⅙ recipe
Calories per serving: 187
Macros: Carbohydrates: 31g; Fiber: 5.3g; Protein: 9.3g; Fat: 3.5g

ROASTED PUMPKIN AND GARLIC SOUP

PAREVE

Prep time: 10 minutes | Cook time: 40 minutes | Total time: 50 minutes

Yield: 4 servings

Delicious, comforting, healthy, and packed with taste. Roasting the pumpkin together with the garlic gives the soup a depth of flavor and gentle sweetness. You can make a big batch and freeze it.

Ingredients

- 1½-pound (680g) pumpkin, chopped into larger pieces
- 2 carrots, roughly chopped
- 2 onions, roughly chopped
- 1 tablespoon + 1 teaspoon olive oil, divided
- 1 large garlic head
- 3 cups (720ml) vegetable stock (or water)
- 1 teaspoon dried rosemary
- ½ teaspoon turmeric
- 2 tablespoons apple cider vinegar
- Salt and pepper to taste

Variations

- Add fresh or powdered ginger and chili for a spicy kick.
- Serve the soup with a dollop of Greek yogurt or cottage cheese to boost the protein.
- Add zucchini, parsnips, or celery to increase micronutrient content.

Tools

- Aluminum foil
- Cutting board
- Immersion blender
- Kitchen scale
- Large pot
- Measuring cups and spoons
- Rimmed baking sheet
- Sharp knife
- Stock pot (4 liter)
- Vegetable peeler

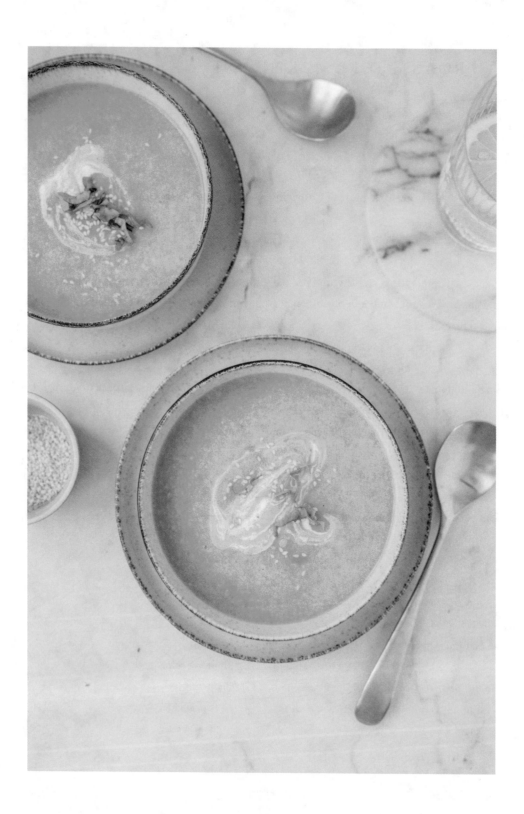

Instructions

1. Preheat the oven to 400°F (200°C).

2. Place chopped pumpkin, carrots, and onions on a large baking sheet and toss with a tablespoon of olive oil. Generously season with salt and pepper.

3. Remove the top ¼ to a ½ inch from the top of the garlic bulb and then peel off the outer papery layer of skin. Place the bulb on a piece of aluminum foil, drizzle with a teaspoon of olive oil, and wrap in the foil. Place the garlic packet on the baking sheet with the vegetables.

4. Transfer the baking sheet to the oven to roast until the vegetables are fork-tender and golden, around 30 to 40 minutes.

5. Transfer the roasted vegetables, along with any juices, to a stock pot set over medium heat.

6. Squeeze the roasted garlic straight into the pot and discard the skin.

7. Pour in the vegetable stock and add the rosemary and turmeric. Bring the soup to a boil and cook for 4 to 5 minutes to allow the flavors to meld together.

8. Allow to cool for 5 minutes, then puree the soup with an immersion blender.

9. Stir the apple cider vinegar through the blended soup and add salt and pepper to taste. Serve immediately.

Serving size: ¼ recipe
Calories per serving: 146
Macros: Carbohydrates: 25g; Fiber: 3.1g; Protein: 2.9g; Fat: 5.3g

ROASTED THREE MUSHROOM AND LEEK STEW

PAREVE

Prep time: 10 minutes | Cook time: 30 minutes | Total time: 40 minutes

Yield: 4 servings

This comforting roasted mushroom stew is creamy, earthy, and light. In this recipe, roasting the mushrooms enhances their taste, and arrowroot powder thickens to creates a silky texture.

Ingredients

- 1 pound (454g) cremini mushrooms
- 1 pound (454g) shiitake mushrooms
- 1 pound (454g) oyster mushrooms
- 1 tablespoon + 1 teaspoon olive oil, divided
- 1 tablespoon water
- 3 leeks, sliced
- 4 garlic cloves, minced
- 2 teaspoons dried thyme
- 5 cups (1170ml) vegetable stock
- 2 cups (67g) fresh kale, thinly sliced
- 2 tablespoons arrowroot powder
- 2 tablespoons cold water
- Salt and pepper to taste

Variations

- Replace the leeks with caramelized onions for a sweeter taste.
- Add white beans or chickpeas to the soup for extra protein.
- Add shredded Cheddar cheese or a dollop of sour cream for a dairy option.

Tools

- Cutting board
- Immersion blender (optional)
- Kitchen scale
- Measuring cups and spoons
- Rimmed baking sheet
- Sharp knife
- Small bowl
- Spatula
- Stock pot (4 liter)
- Vegetable peeler

Instructions

1. Preheat the oven to 400°F (200°C).

2. Place mushrooms on a rimmed baking sheet and toss with a tablespoon of olive oil and a pinch of salt. Roast in the oven until they are a deep golden brown color, around 15 to 20 minutes.

3. In the meantime, heat the remaining teaspoon of olive oil and tablespoon of water in a stock pot over medium heat.

4. Add the leeks and season with a pinch of salt and pepper. Cook, stirring occasionally, until the leeks are soft, around 6 to 8 minutes.

5. Add the garlic and continue cooking for another 1 to 2 minutes.

6. Add the dried thyme and vegetable stock, and bring the stock to a boil.

7. Remove the mushrooms from the oven and roughly chop. Add them to the pot along with the kale, then let everything cook together for another 4 to 5 minutes.

8. In a small bowl, mix the arrowroot starch and 2 tablespoons of cold water to create a "slurry." Add the arrowroot slurry to the mushroom stew.

9. Cook, stirring occasionally, until the arrowroot starch thickens the stew, another 2 to 3 minutes. Taste and adjust the seasoning with more salt and pepper, if needed.

10. Serve immediately, or blend smooth first.

Serving size: ¼ recipe
Calories per serving: 190
Macros: Carbohydrates: 29g; Fiber: 4.6g; Protein: 9.8; Fat: 6.3g

SLOW COOKER CHICKEN SOUP

MEAT

Prep time: 15 minutes | Cook time: 8 hours | Total time: 8 hours 15 minutes

Yield: 6 servings

This classic and comforting chicken soup feels like a hug in a bowl. You can throw everything in the slow cooker in the morning, and you'll have a filling and nutritious meal to enjoy that evening. It is packed with protein from the chicken and micronutrients from all the vegetables.

Ingredients

- 2 onions, chopped
- 4 carrots, diced small
- 2 parsnips or turnips, diced small
- 3 celery stalks, sliced thin
- 5 garlic cloves, minced
- 1½ pounds (680g) chicken breasts, halved
- 1 bay leaf
- 1 teaspoon dried oregano
- 1 teaspoon dried rosemary
- ½ teaspoon dried thyme
- ½ teaspoon paprika
- 4½ cups (1066ml) water
- ½ cup (30g) fresh parsley, chopped
- 2 lemons, cut into wedges
- Salt and pepper to taste

Variations

- Replace the chicken breast with chicken thighs or turkey breasts.
- Use any vegetables that you like or are in season.
- Add canned green chilies, or greens like spinach or kale.
- Add ½ cup of pasta or sliced baby potatoes.
- Replace the spices in the soup with 3 tablespoons of white miso for an extra umami taste.
- Add matzo balls before serving.

Tools

- Cutting board
- Kitchen scale
- Sharp knife
- Slow cooker
- Vegetable peeler

Instructions

1. Add onions, carrots, parsnips, celery, and garlic to the slow cooker.

2. Add the chicken on top of the vegetables and season with salt and pepper.

3. Add the bay leaf, oregano, rosemary, thyme, paprika, and water. Top with the lid and set the slow cooker to low. Leave to cook for 8 hours.

4. Once the soup is done, remove the chicken pieces and slice into thin strips. Return the chicken to the slow cooker and adjust the seasoning with more salt and pepper, if needed.

5. Serve the soup warm along with chopped parsley and lemon wedges.

Serving size: ⅙ recipe
Calories per serving: 225
Macros: Carbohydrates: 13g; Fiber: 3.6g; Protein: 30g; Fat: 4.1g

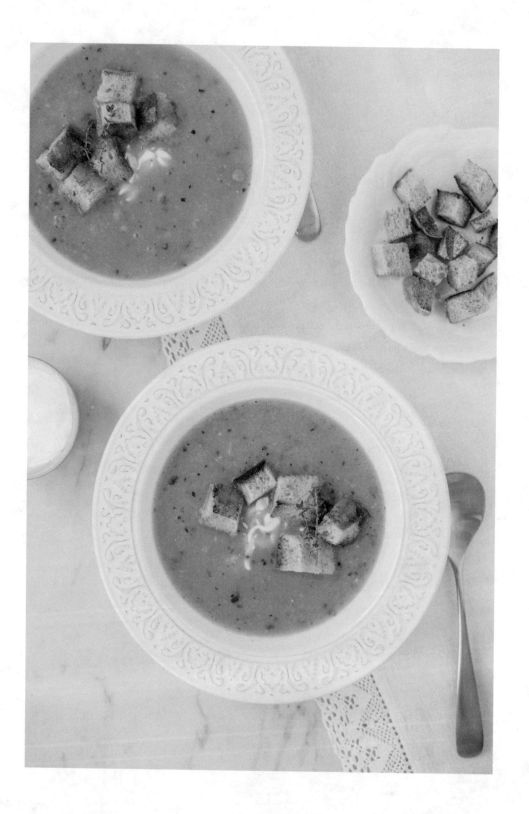

SPLIT PEA, CELERY, AND ZUCCHINI SOUP WITH FRESH LEMON JUICE

PAREVE

Prep time: 15 minutes | Cook time: 1 hour | Total time: 1 hour 15 minutes

Yield: 6 servings

This soup is inspired by a soup I found during my first weeks living in France in 2020, at a popular food store called Picard, which specializes in gourmet frozen food products. Unlike other split pea soups that can be thick and stodgy, this soup is fresh and light. The added zucchini, celery, and lemon lighten and brighten.

Ingredients

- 1 tablespoon water
- 1 teaspoon olive oil
- 2 medium yellow onions, diced small
- 1 shallot, diced small
- 2 garlic cloves, minced
- 1 bay leaf
- 2 medium zucchini, peeled and diced very small
- 2 celery branches, diced very small
- 1¼ cups (250g) dried split green peas
- 5 to 6 cups water
- 1 vegetable bouillon cube
- 1 to 2 tablespoons fresh lemon juice
- Salt and pepper to taste

Tools

- Cutting board
- Immersion blender (optional)
- Kitchen scale
- Measuring cups and spoons
- Sharp knife
- Stock pot (4 liter)
- Vegetable peeler

Instructions

1. To the 4-liter stock pot set over medium heat, add the 1 tablespoon water and olive oil.

2. Add the onions, shallot, salt, and pepper and sauté for 5 minutes, then add the garlic and continue to cook for another 2 minutes.

3. Add the bay leaf, zucchini, celery, split peas, water, and vegetable bouillon cube. Bring to a boil, then simmer uncovered for 1 hour, or until all the peas are soft.

4. During cooking, check frequently and add up to one more cup of water if it looks too dry.

5. Turn off the heat and add fresh lemon juice, and salt and pepper to taste.

6. Serve immediately, or blend partially or completely first.

Serving size: ⅙ recipe

Calories per serving: 151

Macros: Carbohydrates: 30g; Fiber: 9.6g; Protein: 10g; Fat: 2.1g

VEGETABLE CREAM CHEESE SOUP

DAIRY

Prep time: 10 minutes | Cook time: 30 minutes | Total time: 40 minutes

Yield: 4 servings

Cream cheese is the magic ingredient in this foolproof pureed vegetable soup. The cream cheese gives a luxurious, silky texture, along with a pleasant tang. With only a few ingredients, this soup takes just over half an hour to prepare and is full of micronutrients and fiber.

Ingredients

- 2 tablespoons water
- 1 teaspoon olive oil
- 1 medium yellow onion, diced small
- 1 shallot, diced small
- 3 medium zucchini (700–800g), peeled and medium diced
- 3 medium carrots (250–300g), peeled and medium diced
- 2¾ cups (415ml) water
- 1 vegetable bouillon cube
- 2 tablespoons plain cream cheese
- Salt and pepper to taste

Variations

- Add cinnamon, cumin, and cayenne pepper individually or together to add spice.
- Replace the zucchini and carrots with 1 pound of butternut squash.
- Replace the carrot with a fennel bulb for an aniseed taste.
- Use flavored savory cream cheese, such as garlic and herb.

Tools

- Cutting board
- Immersion blender
- Kitchen scale
- Measuring cups and spoons
- Sharp knife
- Spatula
- Stock pot (4 liter)
- Vegetable peeler

Instructions

1. Place the 2 tablespoons of water and olive oil in a 4-liter stock pot set over medium heat.
2. Add the onion and shallot and sauté until translucent, about 10 minutes.
3. Add the zucchini, carrots, water, and vegetable bouillon cube.
4. Bring to a boil, then simmer uncovered for 30 minutes.
5. Allow to cool slightly, then add the cream cheese and blend.
6. Taste and add salt and pepper, if needed.
7. Serve hot.

Serving size: ¼ recipe
Calories per serving: 108
Macros: Carbohydrates: 16g; Fiber: 4.5g; Protein: 3.4g; Fat: 3.9g

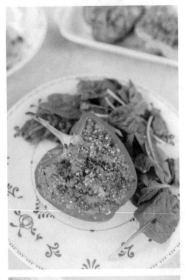

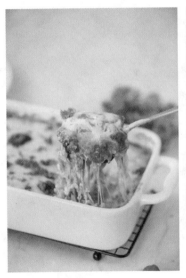

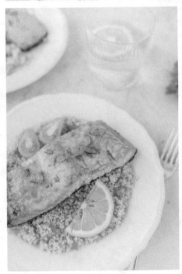

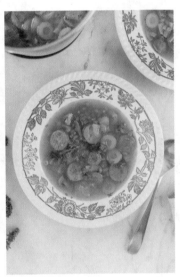

MAIN DISHES

BAKED HERBED CHICKEN BREASTS

MEAT

Prep time: 10 minutes + 1 to 3 hours to marinate for best taste | Cook time: 20 to 25 minutes | Total time: 3 hours 35 minutes

Yield: 6 servings

This marinated and then baked herbed chicken breast recipe is easy to prepare and creates a flavorful main dish for a weekday or holiday meal. The marinade calls for lemon juice and a harissa paste, which brighten and balance the overall taste. It pairs well with whole grains and vegetable sides. It is a perfect recipe for batch cooking.

Ingredients

- 2 pounds (900g) boneless, skinless chicken breasts
- 1 teaspoon salt
- 1 teaspoon black pepper
- 2 garlic cloves, minced
- 1½ tablespoons fresh thyme or rosemary, or a mix of both, chopped
- 2 teaspoons harissa paste
- Juice of 1 lemon

Variations
- Make a simpler marinade with fresh lemon juice and 2 teaspoons olive oil.
- Use different fresh herbs like cilantro, sage, or herbs de Provence.

Tools

- Aluminum foil
- Kitchen scale
- Lidded container or sealable plastic bag
- Measuring cups and spoons
- Rimmed baking sheet

Instructions

1. Pat the chicken breasts dry with paper towels and set aside.

2. Combine the chicken, salt, pepper, garlic, thyme, harissa, and lemon juice in a container with lid or sealable plastic bag, ensuring everything is well-combined and coating the chicken. Leave to marinate for 1 to 3 hours max (the lemon will give the chicken a rubbery texture if left for longer).

3. Preheat the oven to 400°F (200°C) and line a rimmed baking sheet with lightly oiled aluminum foil.

4. Transfer the marinated chicken to the baking sheet and bake in a preheated oven for 20 to 25 minutes.

5. Serve hot or cold.

Serving size: 1 chicken breast
Calories per serving: 160
Macros: Carbohydrates: 1g; Fiber: 0g; Protein: 31g; Fat: 4g

BAKED STUFFED PEPPERS

PAREVE

Prep time: 10 minutes | Cook time: 40 minutes | Total time: 50 minutes

Yield: 12 servings

This baked stuffed pepper recipe features brown rice/quinoa, tempeh, mushrooms, and pine nuts. Each pepper provides plant-based proteins, vitamins, and minerals to provide a balanced meal. The pine nuts add crunch, completing the texture and flavor profile of the recipe. Below are three spice and herb combinations to choose from. This recipe can be a main or a side dish.

Ingredients

- 2 tablespoons water
- 1 medium yellow onion, finely diced
- 3 garlic cloves, minced
- 10 ounces (280g) tempeh, crumbled
- 1 cup (125g) zucchini, diced small
- 2 cups (180g) mushrooms, sliced
- ½ cup (120g) tomato sauce
- Combination of spices (see options below)
- ½ cup (125g) cooked brown rice or quinoa
- ¼ cup (35g) pine nuts
- Salt and pepper to taste
- 6 large bell peppers, cut in half lengthwise and seeds removed
- ¼ cup (15g) freshly chopped parsley

Variations

- Three spice options: oregano and basil; red chili flakes and ground cumin; ginger and smoked paprika.
- For a dairy option, add 1 tablespoon of grated Cheddar cheese to each pepper.
- For another pareve option, replace the tempeh with canned tuna or salmon.
- For a meat option, replace the tempeh with ground turkey or beef.

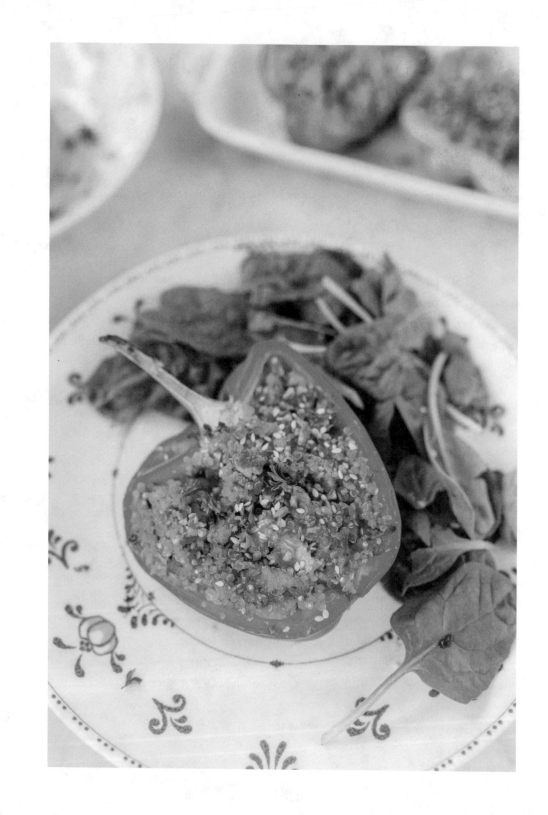

Tools

- Aluminum foil
- Baking dish 9 x 13-inch (33 x 23 cm)
- Cooking oil spray
- Cutting board
- Kitchen scale
- Measuring cups and spoons
- Saucepan
- Sharp knife
- Skillet
- Spatula
- Spoon
- Vegetable peeler
- Wooden spoon

Instructions

1. Preheat the oven to 350°F (180°C), spray the baking dish with cooking oil, and set aside.

2. Heat water over medium heat in a large skillet. Add onion, garlic, and crumbled tempeh. Sauté for about 5 minutes.

3. Add the zucchini, mushrooms, and tomato sauce to the skillet, and cook for about 2 minutes. Season with salt, pepper, and your desired combination of herbs and spices.

4. Add cooked brown rice/quinoa and pine nuts; stir gently to combine, and remove from the heat.

5. Place the bell pepper halves onto the prepared baking dish.

6. Carefully fill each bell pepper with the vegetable mixture. Cover with aluminum foil.

7. Place the dish on the center rack and bake for 25 to 30 minutes. Remove the foil and bake for a further 5 to 10 minutes.

8. Allow the bell peppers to cool slightly before serving.

IF SERVING AS A SIDE DISH

Serving size: ½ pepper

Calories per serving: 133

Macros: Carbohydrates: 9g; Fiber: 1.5g; Protein: 8g; Fat: 5.5g

IF SERVING AS A DAIRY DISH

Serving size: ½ pepper

Calories per serving: 148

Macros: Carbohydrates: 9.4g; Fiber: 1.5g; Protein: 10g; Fat:8.5g

BAKED ZOODLES WITH HERBED RICOTTA, SPINACH, AND MARINARA SAUCE

DAIRY

Prep time: 10 minutes | Cook time: 30 minutes | Total time: 40 minutes

Yield: 6 servings

This zucchini "noodle" (i.e., zoodles) bake recipe has a fresh and delicate taste coming from spinach, zucchini, and umami tomato sauce, alongside the decadent taste of herbed ricotta and mozzarella cheese. Using zoodles instead of pasta makes this dish lighter and lower carbohydrate than normal baked pasta recipes.

Ingredients

- 2 medium zucchini
- Salt (or Kosher salt, see note on p43)
- 3 cups (90g) spinach
- 15 ounces (500g) ricotta cheese
- ⅓ cup (75g) egg whites
- 1 teaspoon dried basil
- 1 teaspoon dried oregano
- ½ teaspoon dried parsley
- ½ teaspoon dried dill
- ½ teaspoon garlic powder
- 2 cups (450g) marinara sauce
- 1 cup (225g) shredded mozzarella

Variations

- Add ½ teaspoon chili flakes or cayenne pepper to add heat.

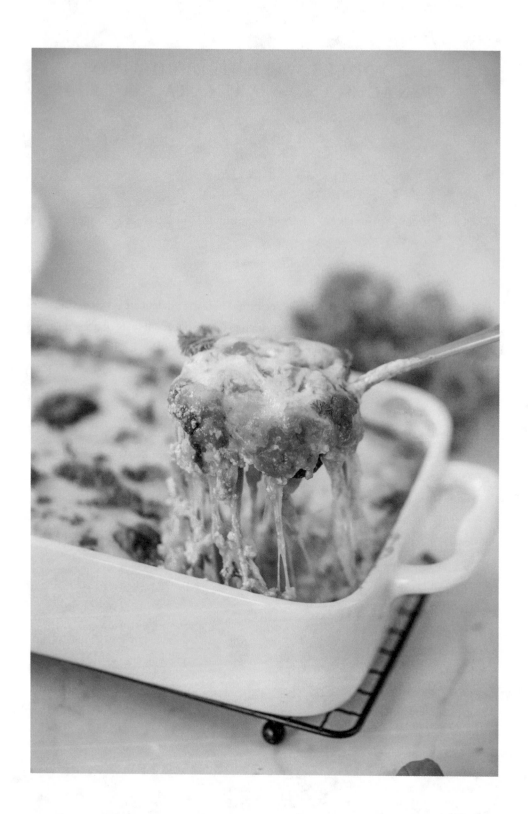

Tools

- Baking dish 9 x 9-inch (23 x 23 cm)
- Cooking oil spray
- Cutting board
- Grater
- Kitchen scale
- Measuring cups and spoons
- Medium mixing bowl x 2
- Microwave safe bowl
- Sharp knife
- Sieve
- Spiralizer
- Spoon

Instructions

1. Preheat the oven to 350°F (180°C) and spray a 9 x 9-inch (23 x 23 cm) baking dish with cooking oil, and set it aside.
2. Spiralize the zucchini into zoodles and trim the long pieces.
3. Toss the zoodles with kosher salt and place in a fine-mesh sieve over a bowl to release excess moisture for about 20 minutes and then squeeze out any excess liquid. This is an essential step or your bake will be too watery.
4. Wilt spinach by placing it with 2 tablespoons water into a microwave-safe bowl. Cover with a lid and microwave on high for 30 seconds to 2 minutes until the leaves wilt. After wilting, squeeze out the excess liquid and set aside.
5. Mix the ricotta, egg whites, basil, oregano, parsley, dill, and garlic powder in a mixing bowl and stir to combine. Set the mixture aside.
6. Assemble in the casserole dish. To layer, start with a quarter of the marinara sauce. Then add half of the spinach, half of the zucchini noodles, half of the ricotta mixture, another quarter of the marinara, and half of the mozzarella cheese. Repeat a second time, finishing with the mozzarella cheese.
7. Bake for 30 minutes or until the cheese is bubbly on top. Allow to cool for 10 minutes before serving.

Serving Size: ⅙ recipe
Calories per serving: 260
Macros: Carbohydrates: 12g; Fiber: 3g; Protein: 19g; Fat: 15g

BEEF AND BROCCOLI

MEAT

Prep time: 10 minutes | Cook time: 15 minutes | Total time: 25 minutes

Yield: 8 servings

This recipe is inspired by Chinese food, which is a staple in American Jewish culture. This dish pairs quick-cooking flank steak with nutritious fresh broccoli florets, and coats everything with a silky sauce of soy, lemon, ginger, and red pepper flakes. Especially delicious served over rice or quinoa.

Ingredients

- 2 pounds (900g) flank steak or sirloin steak, sliced into strips
- ¼ teaspoon salt
- ¼ teaspoon freshly ground black pepper
- 1 tablespoon extra-virgin olive oil
- 2 garlic cloves, minced
- ½ yellow onion, finely chopped
- 2 green onions, thinly sliced
- 4 cups (285g) broccoli florets
- 1 tablespoon cornstarch
- ½ cup (120ml) water
- 1 tablespoon low-sodium soy sauce
- 1 teaspoon lemon juice
- 1 teaspoon fresh ginger, minced
- Pinch of crushed red pepper flakes

Tools

- Colander
- Cutting board
- Kitchen scale
- Large saucepan
- Measuring cups and spoons
- Sharp knife
- Skillet
- Small bowl
- Small whisk
- Spatula

Instructions

1. Season beef strips with salt and black pepper.

2. Heat the oil in a skillet over medium-high heat. Add the beef in a single layer and cook until lightly browned all over, about 3 minutes. Remove from the pan and set aside.

3. Add minced garlic, onion, and green onions to the same pan. Cook for about 1 minute while stirring frequently. Turn off the heat and set it aside.

4. Bring a large pot with salted water to a boil; add broccoli and cook for about 4 to 5 minutes or until tender. Drain well and transfer the broccoli to a clean bowl.

5. In a small mixing bowl, add cornstarch and water and whisk well.

6. Combine soy sauce, lemon juice, ginger, and red pepper flakes in a medium bowl. Incorporate the cornstarch mixture and stir to combine.

7. Add the sauce to the pan with the onion mixture and heat over medium heat.

8. Add broccoli and cook on medium heat for about 3 more minutes or until the sauce thickens. Add beef strips and cook for 2 to 3 minutes while stirring frequently.

Serving size: ⅛ recipe
Calories per serving: 295
Macros: Carbohydrates: 4g; Fiber: 2g; Protein: 32g; Fat: 7g

BEEF AND WHITE BEAN STEW
IN TOMATO BONE BROTH

Prep time: 10 minutes | Cook time: 2 hours | Serves: 8 servings

This beef and white bean stew is slow cooked with marrow bones and passata to create a satisfying, unctuous and comforting main dish. This stew can be made using chuck beef or brisket. Cooking the stew with marrow bones creates a delicious deep tasting, mineral-rich tomato bone broth. A classic Syrian Shabbat dish, this is lighter than cholent, faster to make, and the leftovers taste great. Cooking this dish makes your house smell like cinnamon.

Ingredients

- 2 cups (360g) of dry cannellini beans or great northern beans, soaked overnight and rinsed
- 1 medium yellow onion, diced small
- 2 shallots, diced small
- 1-2 garlic cloves, minced
- 1 lb. (454g) chuck beef or brisket, cubed
- 1 celery stalk, diced small
- 2 marrow bones
- 1 tsp salt
- 1 tsp black pepper
- ½ teaspoon cinnamon
- Cinnamon stick
- 2 tablespoons tomato paste
- 3 cups (700ml) passata

Variations

- Use lamb shank instead of beef
- When short on time, use 2 cans of cooked beans instead of dried to cut the preparation time
- Instead of cooking it on a stovetop, simply brown the onions and beef for 5 minutes and then put everything in a slow cooker on low for 8-12 hours.
- Before serving, add ½ cup fresh coriander leaves, minced

- Add whole eggs to the pot for the final hour of simmering.
- Serve over whole grain: bulgar, quinoa or brown rice.

Tools

- Cutting board
- Large prep bowl
- Cast Iron Dutch Oven or large soup pot
- Knife
- Wooden spoon

Instructions

1. Place the dried beans in a large prep bowl and cover generously with cold water. Cover and leave to soak overnight, then drain and rinse in cold water.
2. Saute the beef, onions, shallot and garlic in a soup pot over medium heat for five minutes, stirring often.
3. Add enough water to cover the meat, then add the passata, marrow bones, white beans, celery, tomato paste, ground cinnamon, cinnamon stick, salt and pepper.
4. Simmer for 2 hours, or until the beans and meat are tender.
5. If after two hours your beans are not soft enough (beans can be finicky sometimes) remove the cooked beef and set aside while you cook the beans until tender. Add the meat back to the soup pot and simmer for 10 minutes or until the meat is warm.
6. Serve warm over your whole grain of choice or fresh bread.

Serving size: ⅛ recipe
Calories per serving: 341
Macros: Carbohydrates: 39.7; Fiber: 8.7; Protein: 32.4; Fat: 7.2

CHICKEN MEATBALLS IN HARISSA TOMATO SAUCE

Prep time: 15 minutes | Cook time: 40 minutes | Total time: 55 minutes

Yield: 4 servings

These chicken meatballs are cooked alongside chickpeas in an aromatic harissa tomato sauce. This is a deeply flavorful and satisfying main dish. Zucchini is added to the meatballs to make them lighter and juicer. Serve alongside rice or couscous.

Ingredients

- 1 small (200g) zucchini
- 1 pound (454g) ground chicken
- 1 egg white (2 tablespoons)
- ¼ cup (15g) chopped fresh coriander leaves
- 2 teaspoons harissa paste, divided
- 2 tablespoons water
- 1 teaspoon extra-virgin olive oil
- 1 large yellow onion, finely chopped
- ½ teaspoon ground turmeric
- ½ teaspoon ground ginger
- 2 garlic cloves, crushed
- 1 can (8 ounces / 240g) diced tomatoes
- 1½ cups (360ml) water
- ¼ teaspoon ground cinnamon
- 1 can (8 ounces / 240g) chickpeas, drained, rinsed
- Steamed couscous or brown rice (optional, for serving)

Variations
- Make with ground turkey.
- Make it spicy by adding cayenne pepper.

Tools

- Cutting board
- Grater
- Kitchen scale
- Kitchen towel
- Measuring cups and spoons
- Plate
- Paper towels
- Sharp knife
- Skillet
- Spatula
- Wooden spoon

Instructions

1. Wash and grate zucchini, then use a clean kitchen towel to squeeze and remove the excess water.
2. Combine ground chicken, grated zucchini, egg white, coriander, and 1 teaspoon harissa in a bowl.
3. Using wet hands, form the mixture into 16 even balls, about 50 grams per ball. Place them on a clean plate.
4. Add water and oil to a skillet set over medium-high heat. Cook meatballs, turning, for 4 to 5 minutes or until browned all over. Transfer the cooked meatballs to a plate lined with paper towels to absorb any excess oil.
5. In the same pan, add onion and sauté for about 5 minutes or until lightly browned. Add turmeric, ginger, and garlic. Cook, stirring, for 30 seconds.
6. Add tomatoes, water, cinnamon, and remaining harissa. Bring to a boil.
7. Add meatballs and chickpeas. Cover and reduce heat to low. Simmer for 30 minutes.
8. Serve immediately, with couscous or rice if desired.

Serving size: 4 meatballs

Calories per serving: 330

Macros: Carbohydrates: 23g; Fiber: 6g; Protein: 31g; Fat: 12g

DEEP DISH CRUSTLESS FLUFFY EGG QUICHE

DAIRY

Prep time: 10 minutes | Cook time: 45 minutes | Total time: 55 minutes

Yield: 12 slices

This quiche is fluffy, creamy, and delicious. It is lighter than most quiches because it is crustless and uses both whole eggs and egg whites, but is still satisfying as it has whole-wheat flour mixed through it. The addition of cottage cheese makes the taste creamy and rich without making it heavy. This quiche is a good choice to serve to a crowd for a dairy meal. It will become one of the recipes you prepare on a regular basis: it's simple to make, pleases most, and can be eaten directly from the oven or over the following days. It works as a main dish for breakfast, lunch, and dinner.

Ingredients

- Vegetable oil or cooking oil spray, for greasing baking dish
- 10 large eggs at room temperature
- 1 cup (220g) egg whites
- ½ cup (65g) semi whole-wheat flour (or gluten-free flour mix)
- 1½ teaspoon baking powder
- 1 teaspoon salt
- 1 teaspoon pepper
- 2 cups (450g) low-fat cottage cheese
- 2½ ounces (70g) shredded cheese (Gruyere, Emmental, or mozzarella)
- 1 red bell pepper, diced
- 2 cups (60g) fresh spinach, chopped

Tools

- Baking dish 9 x 13-inch (33 x 23 cm)
- Cutting board
- Grater
- Kitchen scale
- Large mixing bowl
- Large spoon
- Measuring cups and spoons
- Sharp knife
- Whisk

Instructions

1. Preheat the oven to 350°F (180°C).
2. Oil the baking dish.
3. In a large bowl, whisk the eggs and egg whites.
4. Add flour, baking powder, salt, and pepper and mix well.
5. Add in cottage cheese, shredded cheese, red bell pepper, and spinach and mix evenly.
6. Pour egg mixture into the prepared baking dish.
7. Bake for 45 to 55 minutes.
8. Let cool for 5 to 10 minutes before serving.
9. Cut into 12 pieces.

Serving size: 1 slice
Calories per serving: 152
Macros: Carbohydrates: 8g; Fiber: 1g; Protein: 14.8g; Fat: 6.4g

CURRIED SPLIT YELLOW AND GREEN PEA STEW

PAREVE

Prep time: 20 minutes | Cook time: 50 minutes | Total time: 1 hour 10 minutes

Yield: 4 servings

This curried split yellow and green pea stew is fragrant and has an unctuous texture and taste from peanut butter. The nutritional value of split peas is high, making them a perfect choice for protein-rich plant-based main dishes. The peeled and diced zucchini "disappears" during cooking, while the peppers add a touch of color. Serve alongside rice, bulgur, or quinoa.

Ingredients

- ½ cup + 1 tablespoon (125g) dry split yellow peas
- ½ cup + 1 tablespoon (125g) dry split green peas
- 1 teaspoon coconut oil
- 2 tablespoons water
- 1 medium yellow onion, finely diced
- 3 shallots, minced
- 3 garlic cloves, minced
- 1 teaspoon fresh ginger, minced
- 1 red pepper, diced
- 1 medium zucchini, peeled and diced small
- ½ teaspoon turmeric powder
- 1 teaspoon curry powder
- 1 vegetable bouillon cube

- 1 tablespoon natural smooth peanut butter or almond butter
- 3½ cups (540ml) of water
- 1 teaspoon white vinegar

Variations

- Replace the curry powder with ½ teaspoon of ground cumin and ½ teaspoon of cinnamon.
- Reduce the water and add a 14-ounce (400g) can of crushed tomatoes.
- Use fresh vegetable stock instead of a bouillon cube.
- Add ¼ to ½ teaspoon of cayenne pepper for a spicier stew.

Tools

- Colander
- Cutting board
- Kitchen scale
- Measuring cups and spoons
- Sharp knife
- Skillet
- Spatula

Instructions

1. Rinse and drain the dry split peas, then set them aside.
2. Add coconut oil and 2 tablespoons of water to a skillet set over medium heat. Add diced onion, shallots, minced garlic, and ginger and sauté for about 4 to 5 minutes.
3. Add pepper, zucchini, turmeric, and curry powder and sauté for another minute.
4. Add in rinsed split peas, vegetable bouillon cube, peanut butter, and 3½ cups water. Cover the pot with a lid and bring to a boil.
5. Reduce the heat to low and simmer, partially covered, for 45 to 50 minutes or until peas have softened to your desired consistency.
6. Remove from the heat and stir in white vinegar to brighten the overall taste.

Serving size: ¼ recipe
Calories per serving: 220
Macros: Carbohydrates: 38g; Fiber: 12g; Protein: 14g; Fat: 6g

EGG NOODLES WITH COTTAGE CHEESE AND SOUR CREAM

DAIRY

Prep time: 1 minute | Cook time: 6 minutes | Total time: 7 minutes

Yield: 1 serving

This recipe is a macros balanced version of a classic Jewish comfort recipe. Pasta—like any carbohydrate—is good for us when eaten in an appropriate portion size, and in balance with protein and fat. As a single-serving portion, this dish resets our perception of what a serving of pasta looks like, and how it feels in our stomach. Serve with steamed greens or any crunchy fresh vegetable.

Ingredients

- 56g extra-wide dry egg noodles (tagliatelle pasta)—approximately ½ cup
- ¾ cup (170g) 2% low-fat cottage cheese
- 1 tablespoon sour cream
- ¼ teaspoon salt, to taste
- ½ teaspoon pepper, to taste
- Sliced fresh vegetables to serve alongside (optional)

Variations

- Add ½ teaspoon brown sugar or maple syrup for a touch of sweetness.

Tools

- Kitchen scale
- Large saucepan
- Measuring cups and spoons
- Wooden spoon

Instructions

1. Cook egg noodles in a large pot of salted boiling water, according to packet instructions.

2. Drain the cooked noodles and return them to the same pot.

3. Stir the cottage cheese through the hot noodles, until well coated.

4. Add sour cream and season with salt and pepper.

5. Serve immediately.

Serving size: full recipe

Calories per serving: 350

Macros: Carbohydrates: 48g; Fiber: 2g; Protein: 35g; Fat: 6g

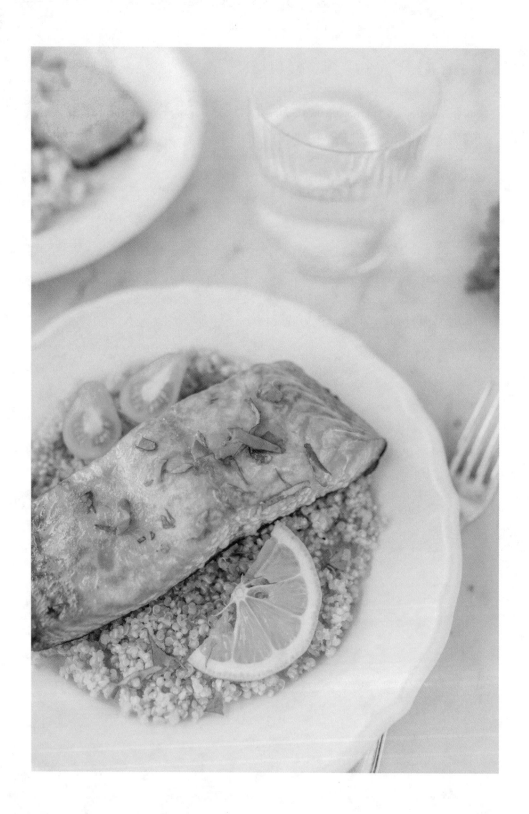

GLAZED SALMON: TWO WAYS

PAREVE

Prep time: 5 minutes | Cook time: 15 to 20 minutes | Total time: 25 minutes

Yield: 4 servings

Salmon is always delicious, even if you don't do anything more than season it with salt, pepper, and fresh lemon juice. When you want an extra-special salmon, here are two glazes that work beautifully baked and pan seared. The first is a Dijon mustard, honey, and apple cider vinegar glaze. The second is a miso and maple glaze. Each creates a unique baked salmon recipe that will please you and your guests from the first bite. An added bonus is this recipe comes together in less than thirty minutes!

Ingredients

- 4 (4-ounce / 140g) wild salmon fillets

For Dijon mustard, honey, and apple cider vinegar glaze:

- 2 tablespoons Dijon mustard
- 1 tablespoon apple cider vinegar
- 1 teaspoon honey
- ½ teaspoon chili powder
- Salt and pepper to taste

For miso and maple glaze:

- 1 teaspoon maple syrup
- 1 tablespoon white miso paste

- 2 tablespoons rice wine vinegar
- 1 teaspoon low-sodium soy sauce
- ¼ teaspoon sesame oil
- 1 garlic clove, minced (optional)

Variation

- Pan sear for 3 minutes per side (or according to personal taste) before adding the glaze. Cook for one minute more, then serve.

Tools

- Aluminum foil
- Kitchen scale
- Measuring cups and spoons
- Rimmed baking sheet
- Small bowl
- Small whisk

Instructions

1. Preheat the oven to 375°F (190°C). Line a baking sheet with foil and grease with vegetable oil.
2. Whisk together preferred sauce ingredients in a small bowl.
3. Place salmon fillets onto the prepared baking sheet. Spread glaze mixture evenly over the fillets. Bake for 15 to 20 minutes or until the salmon flakes with a fork.

WITH DIJON MUSTARD, HONEY, AND APPLE CIDER VINEGAR GLAZE

Serving size: 1 salmon fillet

Calories per serving: 260

Macros: Carbohydrates: 3g; Fiber: 0.4g; Protein: 30.7g; Fat: 12g

WITH MISO AND MAPLE GLAZE:

Serving size: 1 salmon fillet

Calories per serving: 261

Macros: Carbohydrates: 2.5g; Fiber: 0.5g; Protein: 30.8g; Fat: 12.5g

HONEY SESAME CHICKEN WITH GREEN BEANS

MEAT

Prep time: 15 minutes | Cook time: 15 minutes | Total time: 30 minutes

Yield: 4 servings

An easy stovetop recipe, inspired by American Chinese food, with bite-size pieces of chicken breast and crunchy green beans in a slightly sweet umami honey and soy sesame sauce. Especially delicious served over rice or quinoa.

Ingredients

- 1 pound (454g) boneless, skinless chicken breast
- 1 teaspoon extra-virgin olive oil + 1 tablespoon water
- 3 cups (370g) of green beans
- Pinch of salt and pepper

For the sesame honey sauce:
- 1 tablespoon honey
- ¼ cup (60ml) low-sodium chicken broth or water
- ¼ cup (60ml) soy sauce
- 1 teaspoon sesame oil
- 1 teaspoon lemon juice or apple cider vinegar
- 1 garlic clove, minced

- 2 teaspoons cornstarch
- 1 tablespoon cold water
- 1 tablespoon sesame seeds

Tools

- Cutting board
- Kitchen scale
- Measuring cups and spoons
- Plate
- Sharp knife
- Skillet
- Small bowl x 2
- Small whisk
- Spatula

Instructions

1. In a small bowl, whisk together the sesame honey sauce ingredients: honey, chicken broth, soy sauce, sesame oil, lemon juice, and garlic.

2. In a separate small bowl, whisk the cornstarch with a tablespoon of cold water and set aside.

3. Cut chicken breast into 1-inch (2½cm) pieces. Season with salt and pepper and set aside.

4. Add olive oil and water to a large skillet and heat over medium heat.

5. Add the green beans and sauté for about 2 to 3 minutes or until vegetables are tender. Gently stir from time to time.

6. Transfer the cooked green beans to a clean plate. Cover to keep warm.

7. In the same pan, add the chicken pieces in a single layer. Do this procedure in batches if your pan is not large enough. Cook for 3 to 4 minutes, turning frequently until all sides are browned and the pieces are cooked through.

8. Return the green beans to the pan with the chicken and cook for 2 more minutes.

9. Pour the honey-sesame dressing over the chicken and green beans. Cook for about 20 to 30 seconds.

10. Next, add the cornstarch mixture and bring to a boil. Cook for 1 more minute on low heat until the sauce thickens.

11. Top with toasted sesame seeds and serve.

Serving size: ¼ recipe
Calories per serving: 220
Macros: Carbohydrates: 13.8g; Fiber: 2.3g; Protein: 25.6g; Fat: 8.3g

INDIVIDUAL MUFFIN TIN
TURKEY MEATLOAF

Prep time: 10 minutes | Cook time: 15 to 20 minutes | Total time: 30 minutes

Yield: 8 meatloaves

This simple turkey meatloaf recipe is easy to make, moist, flavorful, and delicious. This will be one of the recipes in your weekly meal plan. Perfect for batch cooking, cooking the meatloaf mix in small portions makes this an easily transportable option for lunch.

Ingredients

- 1¼ pound (570g) ground turkey
- ⅓ cup (30g) plus 2 tablespoons matzo meal, oats, or almond flour (gluten-free option)
- 2 eggs
- 1 medium onion, diced
- ¼ cup (60g) ketchup
- ¼ teaspoon salt, to taste
- ½ teaspoon pepper, to taste

Tools

- Cutting board
- Kitchen scale
- Measuring cups and spoons
- Medium mixing bowl
- Muffin tin
- Sharp knife

Variations
- Add heat: Add a dash of sriracha to the ketchup.
- BBQ flavor: Swap out the ketchup for BBQ sauce.
- Place all the mixture into a lined loaf tin, for a typical meatloaf presentation.

Instructions

1. Preheat the oven to 400°F (200°C).

2. In a medium bowl combine turkey, matzo meal, eggs, onion, ketchup, and salt and pepper.

3. Mix with your hands until just fully combined; do not overmix.

4. Roll into balls (about 100 grams each) and press into muffin pan holes.

5. Bake for about 15 minutes, until cooked through and lightly browned.

6. Serve immediately, or leave to cool and store in a container in the refrigerator.

Serving size: 1 meatloaf
Calories per serving: 186
Macros: Carbohydrates: 3.8g; Fiber: 1g; Protein: 21.7g; Fat: 9.5g

LEMON BAKED WHITE FISH

Prep time: 10 minutes | Cook time: 12 minutes | Total time: 22 minutes

Yield: 4 servings

A simple, delicious, and mild lemon-garlic baked white fish recipe that is ready in twenty minutes. Combine this with a fresh salad and carbohydrate of your choice.

Ingredients

- 2 garlic cloves, minced
- 2 teaspoons extra-virgin olive oil (or butter or vegan butter), divided
- 1 lemon
- 1½ pounds (680g) white fish fillets (tilapia, cod, haddock, halibut)
- ¼ teaspoon salt
- ¼ teaspoon ground black pepper
- Freshly chopped parsley for garnish (optional)

Tools

- Baking dish 9 x 13-inch (33 x 23 cm)
- Cutting board
- Kitchen scale
- Measuring cups and spoons
- Sharp knife
- Skillet
- Small bowl
- Spatula

Instructions

1. Preheat the oven to 400°F (200°C) and lightly grease a glass baking dish with olive oil.
2. Add 1 teaspoon of olive oil to a skillet and heat over medium-high heat. Add minced garlic and sauté for about 2 minutes.

3. Cut the lemon in half. Squeeze one half and pour the juice into a small mixing bowl. Thinly slice the other half.

4. Arrange the lemon slices on the prepared baking dish.

5. Carefully arrange the fish fillets on top of the lemon slices. Season with salt and pepper and drizzle with lemon juice and the remaining olive oil.

6. Bake the fish fillets for about 10 to 12 minutes—adjust according to type and size of fillet used. When it flakes easily it means it is cooked through.

Optional: serve with freshly chopped parsley on top.

Serving size: ¼ recipe
Calories per serving: 245
Macros: Carbohydrates: 2.9g; Fiber: 1g; Protein: 34.9g; Fat: 9.6g

MIX-AND-MATCH BALANCED MACROS PLATE TEMPLATE

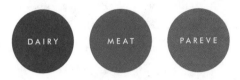

Prep time: 5 minutes

Yield: 1 serving

We often put together meals without recipes, using ingredients as building blocks. Eating a macros-friendly meal is simple. Using this template will help you learn by doing. This balanced meal template includes protein, carbohydrates, fat, and micronutrients and you can simply mix and match to create many different meals. Track individual food items and quantities to get specific calorie and macros breakdown.

Ingredients

Greens and non-starchy vegetables, 1 cup of any of the following, or mix and match:

- Greens (arugula, spinach, kale, lettuces)
- Cucumbers
- Celery
- Cauliflower, blanched
- Broccoli, blanched
- Green beans, raw or blanched
- Bell peppers, raw or blanched

Protein, 1 of the following:

- 120 grams of tuna, packed in water
- 120 grams of cooked chicken breast
- 120 grams of cooked turkey
- 100 grams of cooked tofu

Carbohydrates, 1 of the following:

- 80 grams of cooked quinoa
- 80 grams of cooked pasta
- 80 grams of cooked brown or white rice
- 80 grams of cooked lentils
- 100 grams of cooked sweet potatoes

Fat, 1 of the following

- 30 grams of avocado
- 1 tablespoon of olive oil/avocado oil/walnut oil
- 1 teaspoon of nuts (walnuts, almonds, cashews, macadamia)
- 30 grams of olives

Optional:

- Any vinegar
- Fresh lemon juice
- Fresh herbs
- Garlic or sliced green onions

Tools

- Cutting board
- Kitchen scale
- Measuring cups and spoons
- Mixing bowl
- Sharp knife
- Spoon
- Vegetable peeler

Instructions

1. To a mixing bowl, add one cup of your chosen green or non-starchy vegetable.
2. Add your chosen source of protein.
3. Add your chosen carbohydrate.
4. Add your chosen fat.
5. Dress with vinegar, lemon juice, garlic, or sliced green onion.
6. Mix to combine, and serve.

Serving size: full recipe

Calories per serving: approximately 400

Macros: Track individual food quantities to get specific calorie and macros breakdown that works for you.

MUSHROOM AND BARLEY
STEW WITH SAUSAGE

MEAT

Prep time: 15 minutes | Cook time: 1 hour | Total time: 1 hour 15 minutes

Yield: 6 servings

This barley-based dish makes a satisfying main dish. This stew pairs barley with kosher sausages, fresh vegetables, and a mix of mushrooms. The combination of meaty, plump portobellos along with savory, flavor-rich white button and cremini mushrooms is delicious. Toasted sunflower seeds and freshly chopped parsley provide a contrasting crunch and warm, aromatic finish.

Ingredients

- 8 ounces (220g) turkey sausages
- 1 teaspoon olive oil
- 2 tablespoons water
- 1 medium yellow onion, thinly diced
- 1½ cups (150g) white button mushrooms, sliced
- 1½ cups (150g) cremini mushrooms, sliced
- 2 portobello mushrooms, sliced
- 1 medium carrot, thinly sliced
- 1 large celery stalk, thinly sliced
- 2 garlic cloves, minced
- 1 bay leaf
- ½ teaspoon thyme
- ½ cup (100g) uncooked pearl barley

- 2½ to 3 cups (600–720ml) water or broth of your choice, depending on the consistency you prefer for your stew
- ¼ teaspoon salt
- ½ teaspoon black pepper
- ⅓ cup (20g) freshly chopped parsley

Variations

- Use meat-free sausages for a vegan option.
- Use beef or turkey sausages.

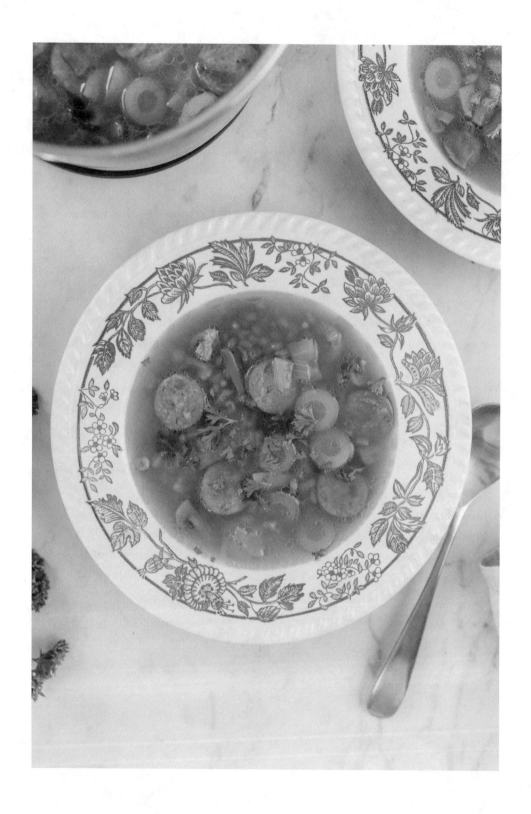

Tools

- Cutting board
- Kitchen scale
- Measuring cups and spoons
- Sharp knife
- Skillet with lid
- Spatula
- Vegetable peeler

Instructions

1. Remove the casings from the sausages.
2. Heat olive oil and 2 tablespoons of water in a skillet over medium heat.
3. Slice the sausages into chunks and cook for 6 to 8 minutes, until browned all over and cooked through. Remove from the pan and set aside.
4. To the same pan (resist the urge to clean it) add onion, mushrooms, sliced carrot, celery, garlic, bay leaf, and thyme and sauté for 5 minutes.
5. Stir in barley and 1½ cups water/broth and season with salt and pepper. Bring to a boil, cover the pan with a lid, and continue cooking on low heat for about 40 to 45 minutes. Check occasionally during cooking, and add more water/broth if it looks too dry.
6. When the stew is done, discard the bay leaf and add the cooked sausage to rewarm it.
7. Serve immediately with parsley on top.

Serving size: ⅙ recipe
Calories per serving: 222
Macros: Carbohydrates: 27g; Fiber: 15g; Protein: 14g; Fat: 8g

NO FUSS VEGETARIAN LASAGNA

DAIRY

Prep time: 20 minutes | Cook time: 1 hour | Total time: 1 hour 20 minutes

Yield: 9 to 12 pieces

This vegetarian lasagna is simple and quick to put together. It is a higher protein and lower fat lasagna and enjoyed by all. You can use homemade tomato sauce and lentils, but it is faster to use labor-saving canned versions. Any tomato sauce can be used, from basic tomato and basil, to spicy Arrabbiata sauce, to a chunky vegetable and tomato sauce. This is a great dairy main dish for a crowd.

Ingredients

- 4 pounds (1.8kg/1870g) tomato sauce
- 14 ounces (400g) tomato pulp
- 7 ounces (200g) low-fat cottage cheese
- 5 ounces (140g) unsweetened plain low-fat Greek yogurt
- 9 ounces (255g) cooked lentils
- 16 ounces no-boil lasagna noodles
- 5 ounces (140g) low-fat cheese, grated
- Add spices to taste: cilantro, oregano, dried parsley, and red pepper flakes

Variations

- Add cooked spinach or mushrooms, making sure to squeeze out the excess water from the cooked vegetables before adding to the sauce.
- Double the recipe and put one in the freezer.
- Use black beans or cannellini beans instead of lentils.
- Bake a day ahead to enhance the flavor.

Tools

- Aluminum foil
- Baking dish 9 x 13-inch (33 x 23 cm)
- Cooking oil spray
- Grater
- Kitchen scale
- Ladle
- Large mixing bowl
- Measuring cups and spoons
- Spatula

Instructions

1. Preheat the oven to 375°F (190°C) and grease the lasagna pan with a bit of vegetable oil or some non-stick baking spray.
2. Spread a thin layer of just tomato sauce on the bottom of a baking dish.
3. In a large bowl, mix together the remaining tomato sauce, tomato pulp, cottage cheese, yogurt, and lentils.
4. Add a layer of lasagna noodles.
5. Add a thin layer of sauce and sprinkle grated cheese on top.
6. Repeat steps 4 and 5 until you run out of ingredients.
7. Cover with foil sprayed with nonstick cooking spray. Bake for 45 minutes. Remove the foil. Bake for 15 more minutes.
8. Remove from the oven and allow to cool for 15 to 20 minutes before cutting.

Serving size: ⅑ or 1/12 recipe

IF MAKING 9 SERVINGS:
Calories per serving: 252
Macros: Carbohydrates: 39.6g; Fiber: 7g; Protein: 17.7g; Fat: 2.4g

IF MAKING 12 SERVINGS:
Calories per serving: 189
Macros: Carbohydrates: 30g; Fiber: 5g; Protein: 13.3g; Fat: 2g

ONE PAN TOFU WITH VEGETABLES

PAREVE

Prep time: 10 minutes | Cook time: 20 minutes | Total time: 30 minutes

Yield: 2 servings

This tofu and vegetable dish is an easy plant-based dinner that comes together in less than 30 minutes, and as a one-pan recipe the cleanup is minimal.

Ingredients

- 10 ounces (280g) firm tofu, cut into rectangles
- 1 tablespoon olive oil, divided
- 2 tablespoons cornstarch
- 2 cups (142g) broccoli florets
- 2 cups (130g) cauliflower florets
- 2 carrots, chopped
- 1 red onion, chopped
- 2 tablespoons soy sauce
- 1 garlic clove, minced
- 1 scallion, thinly sliced
- ½ cup (30g) chopped parsley
- Juice of ½ lemon
- Salt and pepper to taste

Variations

- Coat tofu with orange juice, honey, and rosemary for a different flavor profile.
- Use any vegetables that are in season or you already have on hand.
- You can double or triple the amount of tofu and use it to top a salad or crumble it over pasta for added protein.
- If tofu is not your thing, make this with chicken breast pieces.

Tools

- Cutting board
- Kitchen scale
- Measuring cups and spoons
- Parchment paper
- Rimmed baking sheet
- Sharp knife
- Spatula
- Vegetable peeler

Instructions

1. Preheat the oven to 400°F (200°C) degrees and line a rimmed baking sheet with a piece of parchment paper.

2. Toss tofu with ½ tablespoon of olive oil and then coat with cornstarch. Arrange tofu on 1 half of the prepared baking sheet.

3. Toss the broccoli, cauliflower, carrots, and onion with the remaining olive oil and season with salt and pepper to taste. Arrange the vegetables on the other half of the baking sheet.

4. Place the baking sheet in the oven and roast for 10 minutes. After 10 minutes, remove from the oven to cover the tofu with the soy sauce and garlic. Return to the oven for another 10 minutes, or until everything is golden and slightly crisp.

5. Serve, topping the tofu with sliced scallion and the vegetables with fresh parsley and lemon juice.

Serving size: ½ recipe
Calories per serving: 384
Macros: Carbohydrates: 40.1g; Fiber: 7.6g; Protein: 20.3g; Fat: 17.3g

SLOPPY JOES

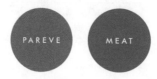

Prep time: 10 minutes | Cook time: 25 minutes | Total time: 35 minutes

Yield: 4 servings

The Sloppy Joe sandwich is an American recipe (hint: one of the ingredients is ketchup), a staple in public school lunchrooms, and a favorite homely dinner or lunch recipe. Here are two Sloppy Joe recipes: a meat version with beef and a "meaty" plant-based version with lentils. Both recipes are delicious served as an open sandwich on top of a toasted hamburger bun or pita bread.

Ingredients

For Sloppy Joes with Lentils:

- 1 tablespoon olive oil
- 1 onion, diced
- 1 carrot, diced
- 1 celery stalk, diced
- 2 garlic cloves, minced
- 1 teaspoon smoked paprika
- 1 teaspoon ground cumin
- ½ teaspoon dry mustard powder
- 1 cup (190g) green lentils, rinsed and drained
- 2 cups (480ml) water
- 1 cup (225g) plain tomato sauce
- 2 tablespoons ketchup

- 1 teaspoon molasses (or maple syrup)
- 1 teaspoon orange zest
- Salt and pepper to taste

Variations

- Add ½ teaspoon cayenne pepper or chili powder to either recipe for a spicier version.
- Instead of ground beef, use ground turkey.
- Instead of bread, serve with brown rice, couscous, or quinoa.

Tools

- Cutting board
- Kitchen scale
- Measuring cups and spoons
- Sharp knife
- Skillet with lid
- Spatula or wooden spoon

Instructions for Sloppy Joes with Lentils

1. Heat olive oil in a skillet over medium heat. Add onion, carrots, celery, and garlic; season with a pinch of salt and pepper. Cook, stirring occasionally, until the vegetables become soft and translucent, around 3 to 4 minutes.

2. Stir in paprika, cumin, and dry mustard; continue cooking for another minute until the spices become fragrant.

3. Add in the lentils, water, and tomato sauce; increase the heat to high and bring the mixture to a boil. Reduce the heat to medium-low and cook, partially covered, until the lentils are cooked and everything thickens up, around 18 to 20 minutes.

4. Uncover and stir in the ketchup, molasses, and orange zest. Continue cooking for another 3 minutes.

5. Taste and add more salt, pepper, and spices to taste.

Ingredients

For Sloppy Joes with Lean Ground Beef:

- 1 pound (454g) lean ground beef
- 1 onion, diced
- 1 carrot, diced
- 1 celery stalk, diced
- 2 garlic cloves, minced
- 1 teaspoon smoked paprika
- 1 teaspoon ground cumin
- ½ teaspoon dry mustard powder
- 1 cup (225g) plain tomato sauce
- 2 tablespoons ketchup
- 1 teaspoon molasses (or maple syrup)
- 1 teaspoon orange zest
- Salt and pepper to taste

Instructions for Sloppy Joes with Lean Ground Beef

1. Heat a frying pan over medium-high heat and add the lean ground beef, and sauté, stirring occasionally, for 4 to 5 minutes, or until the meat is no longer pink. Place in a colander or on a paper towel to drain off the excess fat.

2. In the same unwashed skillet, add onions, carrot, celery, and garlic, and season with a pinch of salt and pepper. Cook, stirring occasionally, until the vegetables become soft and translucent, around 3 to 4 minutes.

3. Stir in paprika, cumin, and dry mustard; continue cooking for another minute until the spices become fragrant.

4. Add in tomato sauce, ketchup, molasses, orange zest, and the cooked beef and heat for 3 minutes.

5. Taste and add more salt, pepper, and spices if desired.

SLOPPY JOES WITH LENTILS:
Serving size: ¼ recipe
Calories per serving: 289
Macros: Carbohydrates: 50.8g; Fiber: 11g; Protein: 12.6g; Fat: 5.4g

SLOPPY JOES WITH LEAN GROUND BEEF:
Serving size: ¼ recipe
Calories per serving: 308
Macros: Carbohydrates: 21.3g; Fiber: 4g; Protein: 25.1g; Fat: 14.4g

THREE BEAN TURKEY CHILI

MEAT

Prep time: 5 minutes | Cook time: 40 minutes | Total time: 45 minutes

Yield: 6 servings

This three bean turkey chili is quintessential cold-weather fare served over rice or a baked potato. This recipe features lean ground turkey, three types of beans, fresh vegetables, and a specific blend of spices that is flavorful without being too spicy.

Ingredients

- 1 teaspoon extra-virgin olive oil
- 4 tablespoons water, divided
- 1 pound (454g) lean ground turkey
- ½ teaspoon salt, divided
- ½ teaspoon ground black pepper, divided
- 1 yellow onion, chopped
- 2 garlic cloves, minced
- ½ cup (130g) canned red beans, drained and rinsed
- ½ cup (130g) canned black beans, drained and rinsed
- ½ cup (130g) canned lentils, drained and rinsed
- ¼ cup (55g) canned diced tomatoes
- ¾ cup (180ml) tomato sauce
- 1 cup (240ml) water
- 1 teaspoon chili powder

- ½ teaspoon cayenne pepper
- ½ teaspoon smoked paprika
- ¼ teaspoon ground cumin
- ¼ cup freshly chopped parsley or cilantro

Tools

- Can opener
- Cutting board
- Kitchen scale
- Measuring cups and spoons
- Serving spoon
- Sharp knife
- Skillet
- Spatula

Instructions

1. Heat the olive oil and 2 tablespoons of water in a skillet over medium heat.
2. Add ground turkey and cook, stirring occasionally, until cooked through and browned. Season with salt and pepper and set aside.
3. In the same skillet, heat 2 tablespoons of water and sauté the chopped onion and garlic until translucent, about 2 to 3 minutes.
4. Add all the beans, diced tomato, tomato sauce, and water to the onions. Season with chili powder, cayenne pepper, paprika, cumin, and salt and pepper to taste.
5. Add the cooked turkey back into the pot and bring the chili to a boil. Reduce heat and allow to simmer uncovered for 30 minutes.
6. Portion the chili into bowls, garnish with fresh parsley and cilantro, and serve warm.

Serving size: ⅛ recipe
Calories per serving: 255
Macros: Carbohydrates: 17g; Fiber: 5g; Protein: 21g; Fat: 11g

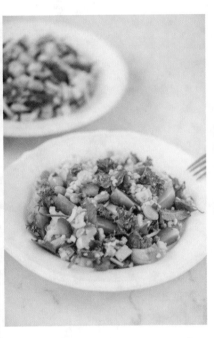
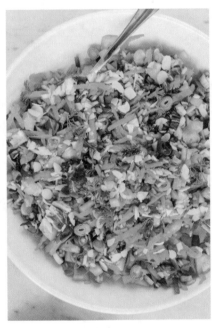
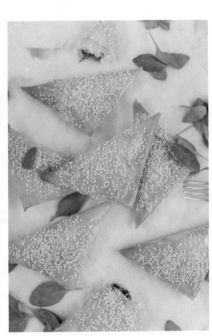

SIDES

"BACON" AND CHEESE TWICE BAKED SWEET POTATOES

DAIRY

Prep time: 15 minutes | Cook time: 1 hour 45 minutes | Total time: 2 hours

Yield: 6 servings

These fake "bacon" and cheese double baked roasted sweet potato halves are a creamy and satiating dairy side dish. They are made with Greek yogurt, butter, milk, a sprinkling of Cheddar cheese, fake "bacon," herbs, and fresh lemon juice.

Ingredients

- 3 large sweet potatoes
- 1 tablespoon light butter, at room temperature
- 1 cup (245g) low-fat Greek yogurt
- 1 teaspoon lemon juice
- 1 cup (240ml) non-fat milk
- ½ medium bell pepper, diced
- ¼ cup fresh chives, chopped
- ½ cup (60g) Cheddar cheese, grated
- ¼ teaspoon dried basil
- ¼ teaspoon dried oregano
- ½ teaspoon garlic powder
- 6 slices of Fakin' Bacon (or another meatless "bacon")

Variations

- Use russet potato instead of sweet potato.

Tools

- Aluminum foil
- Baking dish 9 x 13-inch (33 x 23 cm)
- Cutting board
- Fork
- Kitchen scale
- Measuring cups and spoons
- Sharp knife
- Small bowl
- Spatula
- Spoon

Instructions

1. Preheat the oven to 375°F (190°C). Wrap 3 large sweet potatoes (10 to 12 ounces each) in aluminum foil.

2. Transfer potatoes to the oven and bake for about 1 hour and 30 minutes. When done, a fork or skewer should slide in easily.

3. Remove potatoes from the oven and allow them to cool completely.

4. Use a sharp knife to cut the potatoes in half lengthwise. Gently scrape out the inside of each potato, being careful not to tear the skin.

5. Place the flesh in a mixing bowl and use a fork to mash well. Add in butter, Greek yogurt, lemon juice, and milk. Incorporate bell pepper, half of the chives, and half of the grated Cheddar cheese. Season with dried basil, dried oregano, and garlic powder. Use a spatula to mix.

6. Place the hollowed sweet potato shells in an oven-safe glass baking dish, lightly greased with olive oil.

7. Use a spoon to fill the potato shells with the potato mixture.

8. Crumble one slice of bacon into each potato half.

9. Sprinkle the remaining Cheddar cheese, chives, and "bacon."

10. Transfer the baking dish to the oven. Bake at 350°F (180°C) for 20 to 25 minutes or until the cheese melts and the top of each potato becomes crispy.

Serving size: 1 potato half
Calories per serving: 245
Macros: Carbohydrates: 22.5g; Fiber: 4g; Protein: 10.6g; Fat: 12.5g

BULGUR, FAVA, AND STRAWBERRY SALAD

PAREVE

Prep time: 8 minutes | Cook time: 12 minutes | Total time: 20 minutes

Yield: 4 servings

This seasonal grain salad features two underappreciated ingredients: bulgur wheat and fava beans. Bulgur is cracked wheat made by crushing the blanched hulled kernels of wheat grain. It features regularly in Middle Eastern cuisine, in dishes such as the tabbouleh salad, and can also be used to make porridge. Also known as broad beans, fava is the legume with the highest protein content. They come fresh, frozen, canned, or dried, making them an ideal addition to regular meals. The taste combination offered in this salad is truly unique: cucumber and spinach give a freshness to offset the nuttiness of bulgur. Strawberries give sweet tartness, which can be substituted with tomato when out of season. Fresh mint, cilantro, pepper, and lemon juice envelop everything with zing.

Ingredients

- ¼ teaspoon ground black pepper
- ¼ teaspoon salt

For the dressing:

- ¼ cup (40g) strawberries, blended
- ¼ cup (60ml) lemon juice
- 2 teaspoons walnut oil
- 1 teaspoon maple syrup
- 1 teaspoon chopped cilantro

For the salad:

- 1 cup (182g) coarse bulgur, cooked
- 1½ cups (360ml) water or low-sodium broth
- 1 small red onion, minced
- 1 (15-ounce / 260g) can fava beans, drained and rinsed well

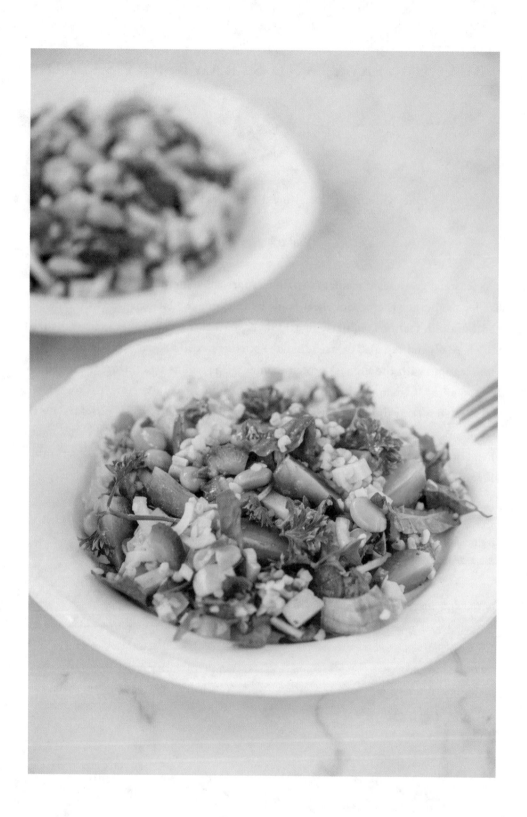

- 1 medium English cucumber, deseeded and diced very small
- 1 cup (30g) finely chopped fresh spinach leaves
- ½ cup (30g) finely chopped fresh parsley
- 1¾ cups (350g) fresh strawberries, quartered, divided
- Salt and ground black pepper to taste

Variations

- For gluten free, use quinoa instead of bulgur wheat.
- In colder months, use cherry tomatoes instead of strawberries.
- Use extra-virgin olive oil instead of walnut oil.
- Switch fava bean to another bean of your choice.

Tools

- Blender
- Can opener
- Colander
- Cutting board
- Kitchen scale
- Large mixing bowl
- Measuring cups and spoons
- Medium saucepan
- Sharp knife
- Small bowl
- Small whisk

Instructions

1. Rinse the bulgur.
2. Bring 1½ cups of low-sodium broth (or water) to a boil in a medium saucepan.
3. Stir in the drained bulgur and allow to boil again.
4. Simmer for 12 minutes. The bulgur should be tender and there should be no liquid left.
5. Remove from the heat and let it stand, covered, for 10 minutes.
6. In a small mixing bowl, add strawberries, lemon juice, walnut oil, maple syrup, cilantro, pepper, and salt for the dressing, and whisk well to combine. Set aside.
7. To a large mixing bowl, add the onion, beans, cucumber, spinach, and parsley for the salad.
8. Drizzle the salad with the dressing and toss gently to coat.
9. Top with the strawberries so they stand out and don't get mashed.
10. Taste and season with salt and pepper if needed.

Serving size: ¼ recipe

Calories per serving: 198

Macros: Carbohydrates: 36g; Fiber: 9g; Protein: 10g; Fat: 3g

CRISPY CHICKPEAS WITH ZUCCHINI OVER HERBED YOGURT

DAIRY

Prep time: 10 minutes | Cook time: 20 minutes | Total time: 30 minutes

Yield: 4 servings

These crispy chickpeas with zucchini over herbed yogurt are savory, crunchy, tangy, and perfectly balanced. You get spice and crunch from the roasted chickpeas, sweetness from the zucchini, tang from the yogurt, and brightness from the herbs. It is also packed with fiber and plant protein from the chickpeas.

Ingredients

- 1 tablespoon olive oil, divided
- 1½ cups (255g) cooked chickpeas (cooked from scratch or canned)
- 1 teaspoon smoked paprika
- 1 teaspoon ground cumin
- 2 small zucchinis, chopped
- 1 cup (280g) low-fat Greek yogurt
- 1 tablespoon lemon juice
- ½ cup (30g) parsley, finely chopped
- ½ cup (5g) fresh dill, finely chopped
- Salt and pepper to taste

Variations

- Replace the chickpeas with white beans.
- Replace the zucchini with eggplant, red peppers, or cauliflower.
- Serve with coconut or soy yogurt for a vegan version.
- Wrap in a whole-grain tortilla or a pita with some extra veggies to make it a full meal.

Tools

- Cutting board
- Kitchen scale
- Measuring cups and spoons
- Parchment paper
- Rimmed baking sheet
- Sharp knife
- Small bowl

Instructions

1. Preheat the oven to 400°F (200°C) degrees and line a rimmed baking sheet with a piece of parchment paper.

2. Add the chickpeas to one half of the prepared baking sheet and toss with ½ tablespoon of olive oil, smoked paprika, and ground cumin. Season with a pinch of salt and pepper.

3. Add the chopped zucchini to the second side of the baking sheet and toss with the remaining olive oil, plus some salt and pepper to taste.

4. Place the baking sheet in the oven and roast until the chickpeas are golden and crunchy and the zucchini is fork-tender and lightly browned, around 15 to 20 minutes.

5. In the meantime, in a small bowl, combine yogurt, lemon juice, and chopped herbs. Season with a small pinch of salt and pepper.

6. Serve the crispy chickpeas and roasted zucchini over the herbed yogurt.

Serving size: ¼ recipe
Calories per serving: 218
Macros: Carbohydrates: 29g; Fiber: 6.4g; Protein: 12g; Fat: 6.1g

GRATED CARROT AND TOASTED BUCKWHEAT GROATS SALAD

PAREVE

Prep time: 20 minutes

Yield: 8 servings

This salad is fresh, sweet, creamy, and crunchy. Carrot salad has to be the least controversial vegetable side dish. The addition of roasted raw buckwheat groats adds a nutty crunch that works well alongside raw vegetables.

Ingredients

- ¼ teaspoon oil (coconut or vegetable oil)
- ½ cup (85g) raw buckwheat groats
- 2.2 pounds (1kg) carrots, grated with food processor

For the dressing:
- ¼ cup (60g) tahini
- ½ cup (120ml) plain oat milk or water
- 2 tablespoons maple syrup
- 3 tablespoons apple cider vinegar
- Salt and pepper to taste

Variations
- Replace ¼ of the carrots with grated purple cabbage or raw beetroot.

- For gluten free, add ½ cup of cooked tricolor quinoa or ½ cup of chopped walnuts.

Tools

- Blender
- Grater
- Kitchen scale
- Large salad bowl
- Measuring cups and spoons
- Salad spoons
- Skillet
- Vegetable peeler
- Wooden spoon

Instructions

1. Heat oil in a skillet over medium heat.

2. Add the buckwheat groats to the pan and toast, mixing occasionally, for 5 to 7 minutes. Set aside.

3. For the dressing, add the tahini, oat milk, maple syrup, apple cider vinegar, and salt and pepper to a blender and blend until smooth. Set aside.

4. Place grated carrots into a large salad bowl.

5. Add the dressing and mix evenly. Taste and adjust the flavor with more vinegar, salt, or maple syrup to taste.

6. Mix in the toasted buckwheat groats right before serving.

Serving size: ⅛ recipe
Calories per serving: 149
Macros: Carbohydrates: 25g; Fiber: 5.1g; Protein: 4g; Fat: 5g

JEWELED RICE

PAREVE

Prep time: 10 minutes | Cook time: 25 minutes | Total time: 35 minutes

Yield: 4 servings

This delicious and colorful dish delights the eyes and mouth. Combining warm rice with a variety of raw vegetables, dried fruits, edamame, and nuts, this vibrant dish has plenty of taste and texture. The edamame is buttery with a hint of sweetness and nuttiness, and you could swap it for frozen peas. The toasted nuts elevate the grain and raw vegetables, adding crunch, flavor, and aroma. A dish that is simple to make yet feels and tastes special.

Ingredients

- 1 cup (170g) carrot, grated
- ½ cup (46g) yellow pepper, thinly sliced
- ½ cup (46g) orange pepper, thinly sliced
- ½ cup (32g) purple cabbage, thinly sliced
- 1 cup (160g) edamame
- ½ cup (52g) of green onion, sliced, green + white parts (or more to taste)
- ½ ounce (14g) dried cranberries, chopped small
- 1 teaspoon lemon zest
- 1 ounce (28g) almonds, roughly chopped and toasted
- 1 cup (165g) cooked brown basmati rice
- 1 teaspoon (5g) vegan butter spread
- Salt and pepper to taste

Variations

- Instead of raw vegetables, lightly steam the vegetables.
- Use any dried fruits or nuts you have on hand for various flavor variations: pecans, pine nuts, pistachios, pumpkin seeds, dried figs, dried cherries, dried apricots, or raisins.
- Replace the rice with quinoa or millet for extra protein and a different texture.
- Replace the edamame with peas.
- Use walnut oil, coconut oil, or real butter instead of vegan butter spread.

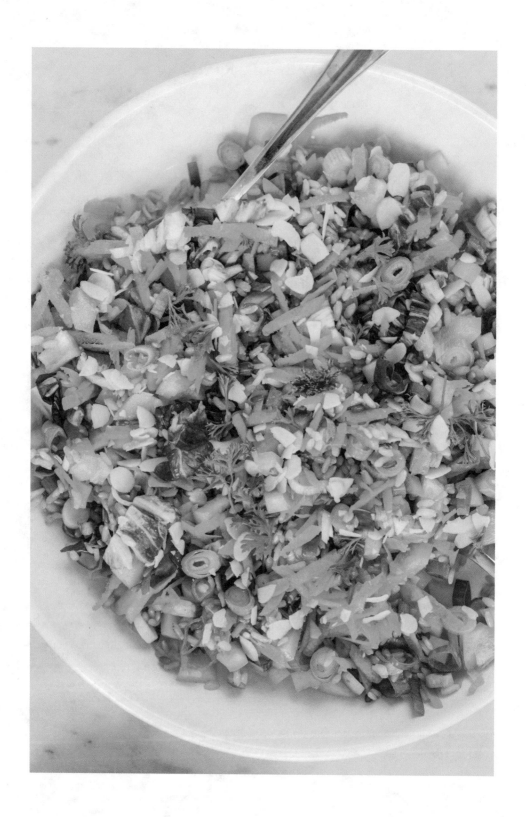

Tools

- Cutting board
- Kitchen scale
- Large salad bowl
- Measuring cups and spoons

- Medium mixing bowl
- Saucepan
- Sharp knife
- Skillet
- Wooden spoon or silicone spatula

Instructions

1. Add the carrots, peppers, cabbage, edamame, onions, cranberries, and lemon zest to a large salad bowl.

2. Toast the almonds in a skillet and set aside.

3. Cook rice according to package directions.

4. Place cooked rice in a prep bowl and combine with butter.

5. Fold rice into a salad bowl with other ingredients.

6. Taste and add salt and pepper to taste.

7. Scatter the toasted almonds on top.

8. Serve immediately.

Serving size: ¼ recipe
Calories per serving: 162
Macros: Carbohydrates: 23.6g; Fiber: 5g; Protein: 5.6g; Fat: 5.5g

LIGHTER POTATO KUGEL

PAREVE

Prep time: 20 minutes | Cooking time: 1 hour | Total time: 1 hour 20 minutes

Yield: 12 pieces

A lighter and fresh take on classic potato kugel, a baked potato casserole. Grated cauliflower and added egg whites make this potato kugel lighter than the classic recipe.

Ingredients

- 2 pounds (900g) russet potatoes (about 8 medium-sized potatoes)
- 1 large yellow onion
- 2 eggs + ¾ cup (180g) egg whites
- ¼ cup + 1 tablespoon potato starch
- ½ teaspoon smoked paprika
- ½ teaspoon salt
- ½ teaspoon black pepper
- 1 tablespoon extra-virgin olive oil
- 4 cups (260g) cauliflower
- Freshly chopped parsley for garnish (optional)
- Freshly chopped chives for garnish (optional)

Tools

- Baking dish 9 x 13-inch (33 x 23 cm)
- Colander
- Cooking oil spray
- Cutting board
- Grater
- Kitchen scale
- Large mixing bowl x 2
- Measuring cups and spoons
- Sharp knife
- Spatula
- Vegetable peeler

Variations
- Replace some, or all, of the potato with sweet potato.

Instructions

1. Preheat the oven to 400°F (200°C). Spray a 9 x 13-inch (33 x 23 cm) baking dish with cooking oil, and set it aside.
2. Peel the potatoes and add them to a large bowl of cold water.
3. Add the eggs, egg whites, potato starch, smoked paprika, salt, and pepper, and oil to a large bowl and stir well to combine.
4. Grate the cauliflower and add to the bowl with the egg mixture.
5. Peel and finely dice the onion, and add to the egg and cauliflower.
6. Drain the potatoes in a colander and rinse under hot running water for 30 seconds to wash away excess starch.
7. Grate the potatoes, and quickly add them to the bowl with everything else. Stir immediately to coat everything and prevent the potatoes from discoloring.
8. Transfer the mixture to the prepared baking dish.
9. Bake for about 50 to 60 minutes.
10. Remove from the oven and set aside to cool for at least 10 minutes.
11. Garnish with freshly chopped parsley and chives before serving.

Serving size: $\frac{1}{12}$ recipe

Calories per serving: 97

Macros: Carbohydrates: 14g; Fiber: 3g; Protein: 6g; Fat: 2g

QUINOA, ROASTED VEGETABLE, AND FETA CASSEROLE

DAIRY

Prep time: 20 minutes | Cook time: 45 minutes | Total time: 1 hour 5 minutes

Yield: 8 servings

This baked quinoa recipe tastes special because it includes three strong flavors: roasted vegetables, feta cheese, and white wine. Enjoy as a main dish or as an accompaniment to fish. Ideal for potlucks or group gatherings, this can be made in advance and is delicious served warm or at room temperature.

Ingredients

- 2 bell peppers, medium diced
- 3 cups of small cauliflower florets
- 1 red onion, thinly sliced into strips
- 3 garlic cloves, minced
- 1 tablespoon olive oil
- 1 cup (185g) quinoa, rinsed
- 2 large handfuls of baby spinach, thinly sliced into strips
- 1 teaspoon herbs de Provence
- ⅓ cup (80ml) dry white wine (regular or non-alcoholic)
- ¾ cup (180g) egg whites, beaten
- Salt and pepper, to taste
- Pinch of red pepper flakes
- 8 ounces (225g) crumbled feta cheese

Variations

- Roast any combination of vegetables: pumpkin, eggplant, zucchini.
- For a non-dairy option, use vegan cheese.

Tools

- Baking dish 9 x 13-inch (33 x 23 cm)
- Kitchen scale
- Measuring cups and spoons
- Saucepan
- Spatula

Instructions

1. Preheat the oven to 400°F (200°C) and lightly oil a 9 x 13-inch (33 x 23 cm) baking dish.

2. Toss the bell pepper, cauliflower, onion, and minced garlic in the baking dish until everything is lightly coated with the oil. Season and spread evenly, then roast in the oven for 25 to 30 minutes.

3. While the vegetables are baking, cook the quinoa according to the directions on the packaging.

4. Remove the roasted vegetables from the oven and stir in the baby spinach, herbs de Provence, and white wine.

5. Add the egg whites and a dash of red pepper flakes, and stir gently until everything is combined.

6. Add the cooked quinoa and fold through until just combined. Make sure the mixture is evenly distributed in the dish.

7. Top with the crumbled feta and bake for another 20 minutes.

8. Turn up the oven temperature to broil for 3 to 5 minutes, until the feta is slightly browned.

9. Serve immediately or later, and refrigerate any leftovers in an airtight container for up to 5 days.

Serving size: ⅛ recipe
Calories per serving: 238
Macros: Carbohydrates: 24g; Fiber: 3g; Protein: 18g; Fat: 8g

RAINBOW VEGETABLE SALAD

PAREVE

Prep time: 15 minutes

Yield: 4 servings

This vibrant salad has bell peppers, cherry tomatoes, purple cabbage, red onion, and a fresh lemon and olive oil dressing. A multicolored dish, this salad is the embodiment of the health principle "eat the rainbow." Different colored fruits and vegetables offer our bodies a variety of vitamins, minerals, and antioxidants.

Ingredients

- 1 pound (454g) sweet multicolored (red, green, yellow, orange) bell peppers
- 1 cup (150g) cherry tomatoes
- ½ small head of purple cabbage
- 1 medium red onion
- 2 tablespoons fresh lemon juice
- 2 tablespoons extra-virgin olive oil
- Pinch of salt and black pepper

Variations

- Add your favorite green leafy vegetable to this to complete the rainbow of colors.
- Swap any of the ingredients for any thinly sliced or shredded vegetable that you enjoy raw.

Tools

- Cutting board
- Kitchen scale
- Large mixing bowl
- Measuring cups and spoons
- Salad spoons
- Sharp knife
- Small mixing bowl
- Small whisk

Instructions

1. Remove the stalks and deseed the bell peppers, then cut into thin strips.

2. Halve the cherry tomatoes and finely shred the purple cabbage.

3. Peel and finely chop the red onion.

4. Add all the vegetables to a large mixing bowl.

5. Combine lemon juice, extra-virgin olive oil, salt, and a pinch of pepper in a small mixing bowl. Whisk the dressing together.

6. Pour the dressing over the salad ingredients and stir well to combine.

Tip: *Refrigerate the salad for a few hours before serving to give the vegetables time to absorb the dressing flavors.*

Serving size: ¼ recipe

Calories per serving: 105

Macros: Carbohydrates: 14g; Fiber: 3g; Protein: 2g; Fat: 5g

ROASTED CABBAGE SALAD WITH WALNUTS AND FETA

DAIRY

Prep time: 10 minutes | Cook time: 15 minutes | Total time: 25 minutes

Yield: 4 servings

This roasted cabbage salad with walnuts and feta is deeply savory, filling, and packed with nutrients.

Ingredients

- 3 teaspoons olive oil, divided
- 1 small head of green cabbage, thinly sliced
- 1 red onion, thinly sliced
- 1 apple, thinly sliced
- 3 tablespoons fresh dill, finely chopped
- 2 teaspoons Dijon mustard
- 2 tablespoons apple cider vinegar
- ¼ cup (30g) walnuts, roughly chopped
- 2 ounces (56g) feta cheese, crumbled
- Salt and pepper to taste

Variations

- Skip the roasting, and serve the cabbage raw as a fresh salad.
- Use thinly sliced or shredded turnips instead of cabbage.
- Use red cabbage or a mix of green and red.
- Use goat cheese and pecans for a different flavor combination.
- Use vegan cheese for a pareve version.

Tools

- Cutting board
- Kitchen scale
- Large mixing bowl
- Large serving dish
- Measuring cups and spoons
- Rimmed baking sheet
- Sharp knife

Instructions

1. Preheat the oven to 400°F (200°C).
2. Toss the cabbage with one teaspoon of olive oil and arrange on a rimmed baking sheet. Season with a pinch of salt and pepper to taste.
3. Place cabbage in the oven to roast until lightly golden brown and crisp around the edges, around 12 to 15 minutes.
4. Remove cabbage from the oven and transfer to a large mixing bowl. Add onion, apple, dill, the remaining extra-virgin olive oil, mustard, and apple cider vinegar; mix well to combine. Season with salt and pepper to taste, remembering that the feta will add saltiness.
5. Transfer salad to a serving dish and top with walnuts and crumbled feta.

Serving size: ¼ recipe

Calories per serving: 230

Macros: Carbohydrates: 27g; Fiber: 8.4g; Protein: 6.7g; Fat: 12g

ROASTED CAULIFLOWER WITH TURMERIC AND PARMESAN CHEESE

DAIRY

Prep time: 5 minutes | Cook time: 15 minutes | Total time: 20 minutes

Yield: 4 servings

Roasted cauliflower is a side dish that works with almost every meal. It is quick, simple, and healthy. When roasting any vegetable, the key to achieving a golden roasted finish is to make sure the pieces are well spread out on the baking sheet.

Ingredients

- 1 head of cauliflower, chopped into thin florets
- 1 tablespoon olive oil
- ½ teaspoon turmeric
- ½ teaspoon garlic powder
- ½ teaspoon salt
- ¼ teaspoon cracked black pepper
- ⅓ cup (30g) Parmesan cheese, grated

Tools

- Cutting board
- Kitchen scale
- Large mixing bowl
- Measuring cups and spoons
- Rimmed baking sheet
- Sharp knife
- Spatula

Variations

- Add smoked paprika and/or chili flakes for a more flavorful version.
- Omit the Parmesan cheese to create a vegan pareve recipe.

Instructions

1. Preheat the oven to 425°F (220°C).

2. In a large bowl, toss cauliflower in olive oil. Sprinkle turmeric, garlic powder, and salt and pepper over cauliflower and toss.

3. Add Parmesan cheese and toss to coat the cauliflower.

4. Transfer to a lightly greased baking sheet and bake for 15 minutes, or until the cauliflower is easily pierced with a fork and golden brown on the edges.

5. Serve immediately.

Serving size: ¼ recipe

Calories per serving: 95

Macros: Carbohydrates: 11g; Fiber: 4g; Protein: 6g; Fat: 4g

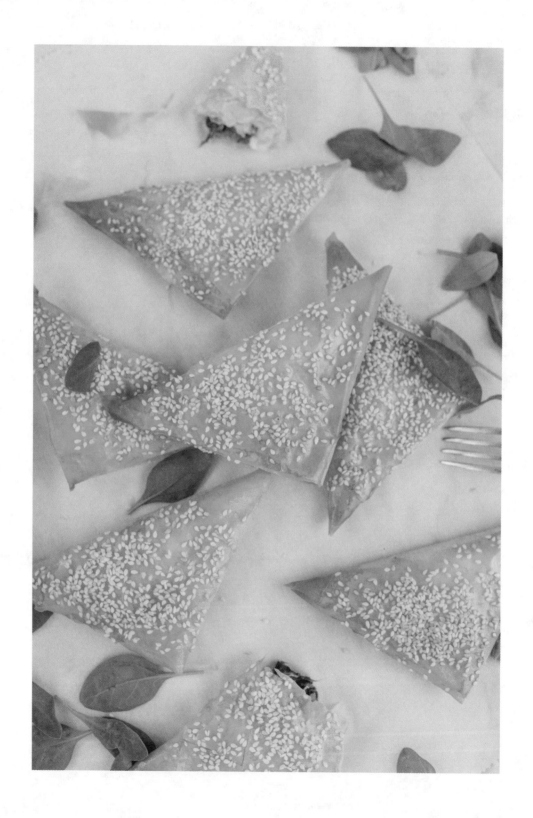

SPINACH AND RICOTTA BOUREKAS

DAIRY

Prep time: 10 minutes | Cook time: 25 minutes | Total time: 35 minutes

Yield: 10 bourekas

These crispy, salty, tangy spinach and ricotta bourekas will be an absolute hit on your dinner table. They are a great party snack or a delicious side.

Ingredients

- 8 ounces (226g) frozen spinach, defrosted overnight
- ½ cup (125g) ricotta cheese
- 1 egg
- 10 phyllo sheets, defrosted overnight
- 3 tablespoons butter, melted (or olive oil)
- 1 to 2 tablespoons sesame seeds, optional
- Salt and pepper to taste

Variations
- Replace the spinach with kale, chard, nettle, or any greens of your choice.
- Replace the ricotta with feta or halloumi.
- Make them dairy-free by using mashed potatoes and sautéed vegetables like mushrooms or peppers.

- Serve with our Roasted Garlic, Yogurt, Turmeric, and Mint Dip (page 37).

Tools

- Cloth
- Colander
- Kitchen scale
- Measuring cups and spoons
- Medium mixing bowl
- Parchment paper
- Pastry brush
- Rimmed baking sheet
- Small bowl
- Spatula

Instructions

1. Preheat the oven to 350°F (180°C) and line a rimmed baking sheet with parchment paper.

2. Place the defrosted spinach in a colander and squeeze out as much water as you can. Transfer spinach to a medium mixing bowl and add in the ricotta and egg; season with salt and pepper and stir to combine.

3. Unroll the defrosted phyllo dough and take one phyllo sheet and fold it in half lengthwise, to make a long, tall rectangle shape. Cover the remaining phyllo with a damp cloth so it doesn't dry out.

4. Lay your folded phyllo sheet on the work surface with the short side in front of you, and lightly brush it all over with melted butter. Dollop a heaping tablespoon of the filling on one of the corners closest to you. Fold the phyllo over the filling and onto itself to form a triangle. Continue folding the phyllo, repeating the triangle shape, until you reach the end of the sheet.

5. Place the phyllo triangle on the prepared baking sheet and repeat the process with all 10 sheets.

6. Brush the triangles with any remaining butter on top. Sprinkle on some sesame seeds, if using, and transfer the phyllo bourekas to the preheated oven. Bake until the phyllo is golden brown and puffy, around 20 to 25 minutes. Leave to cool for a few minutes before serving because the filling will be piping hot.

Serving size: 1 bourekas
Calories per serving: 180
Macros: Carbohydrates: 18g; Fiber: 1.2g; Protein: 5.7g; Fat: 8.5g

SWEET AND SOUR BAKED EGGPLANT

PAREVE

Prep time: 1 hour | Cook time: 1 hour | Total time: 2 hours

Yield: 10 servings

This fragrant, tangy dish features slices of eggplant that are fried and then baked in a zingy tomato and lemon sauce. The sweet-sour taste is perfectly balanced, and the eggplant becomes unctuous in the middle with a wonderful golden crunch on the edges.

Ingredients

- 2 medium eggplants
- ½ teaspoon kosher salt
- 1 medium yellow onion
- 2 tablespoons extra-virgin olive oil
- 1 teaspoon garlic powder
- ½ cup (120ml) tomato paste
- 1½ cups (360ml) of water
- 1 teaspoon sugar
- 2 tablespoons fresh lemon juice
- ½ teaspoon red chili flakes

Variations

- Use zucchini instead of eggplant.

Tools

- Aluminum foil
- Baking dish 9 x 13-inch (33 x 23 cm)
- Colander
- Cooking oil spray
- Cutting board
- Kitchen scale
- Large mixing bowl
- Measuring cups and spoons
- Paper towels
- Plates x3
- Sharp knife
- Skillet
- Small bowl
- Small whisk
- Weight (such as a can)
- Spatula

Instructions

1. Preheat the oven to 300°F (150°C) and spray a 9 x 9-inch (23 x 23 cm) baking dish with cooking oil and set aside.

2. Slice the eggplants into ½-inch thick (1.5cm) rounds and transfer to a colander set over a bowl. Sprinkle the eggplants generously with salt and allow them to sit for 30 to 45 minutes to draw out the excess water.

3. Cover the eggplant with a lid or plate small enough to fit inside the colander, place a weight on top, and set aside for another 30 minutes.

4. Peel and finely dice the onion.

5. Remove the eggplant slices from the strainer and place on a plate lined with paper towels to soak up any excess water.

6. Line another plate or tray with paper towels and set it aside.

7. Add olive oil to a large skillet and heat over medium-high heat.

8. Add eggplant slices to the pan in one layer, taking care not to overcrowd. Fry them for about 2 to 3 minutes per side, flipping when they have developed a deep golden brown color. Tip: shaking the pan occasionally can help prevent sticking.

9. Use a spatula to transfer the fried eggplant slices to the paper towels to absorb excess oil. Repeat with the rest of the eggplant.

10. Return the same pan to medium heat and add the diced onion. Cook until soft, fragrant, and slightly golden, about 5 to 7 minutes. Place it on the bottom of the prepared baking dish and sprinkle it with garlic powder.

11. Layer the fried eggplant slices on top of the onion.

12. In a small bowl, whisk together the tomato paste, water, sugar, lemon juice, and chili flakes. Salt to taste, keeping in mind that the eggplant is already well seasoned. Pour the mixture over the eggplant.

13. Cover the dish with aluminum foil and bake for about one hour.

Serving size: ¹/₁₀ recipe

Calories per serving: 83

Macros: Carbohydrates: 13g; Fiber: 5g; Protein: 2.1g; Fat: 3g

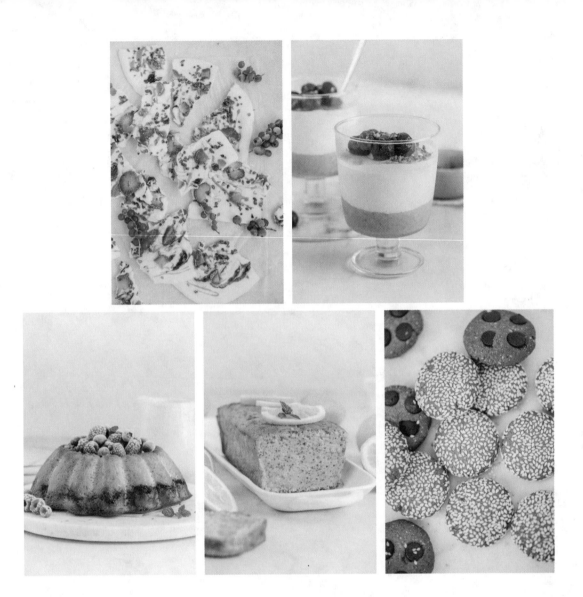

DESSERTS

BAKED HALF APPLE "STRUDEL"

PAREVE

Prep time: 10 minutes | Cook time: 50 minutes | Total time: 1 hour

Yield: 8 half apples

These stuffed baked half apples have the taste profile of apple strudel. The recipe packs delicious and warming flavors into one fruit, nut, and whole-grain dessert. Perfectly spiced with cinnamon and nutmeg, you might want to eat this for breakfast.

Ingredients

- ½ cup (45g) quick-cooking oats
- ¼ cup (24g) almond flour
- 1 tablespoon packed brown sugar
- ½ teaspoon vanilla extract
- ½ teaspoon cinnamon
- ¼ teaspoon nutmeg
- 1 teaspoon stevia
- ¼ teaspoon salt
- 2 tablespoons coconut oil, liquid at room temperature
- 1 tablespoon oat milk
- 4 medium apples
- Juice of ½ lemon
- ½ cup (120ml) water

Variations

- Replace the apples with pears for a different flavor profile.
- Serve it with a dollop of Greek yogurt or vanilla ice-cream.
- Replace the oat milk with rum.
- Use gluten-free oats for a gluten-free version.
- Use quinoa flakes for a kosher-for-Passover version.

Tools

- Aluminum foil
- Cooking oil spray
- Cutting board
- Kitchen scale
- Large mixing bowl
- Measuring cups and spoons
- Rubber spatula
- Sharp knife
- Rimmed baking sheet
- Spoon

Instructions

1. Preheat oven to 375°F (190°C).
2. To a large mixing bowl add rolled oats, almond flour, brown sugar, vanilla, cinnamon, nutmeg, stevia, and a pinch of salt. Mix until combined.
3. Add liquid coconut oil and oat milk. Mix until combined and set aside.
4. Slice the apple in half from stalk to bottom, and remove the core to create a groove. You will end up with two bowl-shaped pieces.
5. Put some coconut oil on your clean hands and lightly coat the cut side of the apples. Stuff 1 tablespoon of the oat mixture into the groove where the core was.
6. Line a baking sheet with aluminum foil and spray with oil.
7. Place the stuffed apples into the lined dish.
8. Squeeze a little fresh lemon juice over each apple.
9. Carefully pour the water around the apples. They should be sitting in the water, not submerged.
10. Cover with another sheet of aluminum foil and bake at 375°F for 20 minutes.
11. Remove the foil cover and bake for another 30 to 40 minutes, until the apples are fork tender.
12. Allow to cool slightly before serving.

Serving size: ½ apple
Calories per serving: 117
Macros: Carbohydrates: 21.4g; Fiber: 3g; Protein: 1.2g; Fat: 4.5g

CHOCOLATE ZUCCHINI CAKE

PAREVE

Prep time: 10 minutes | Cook time: 30 minutes | Total time: 40 minutes

Yield: 8 servings

This delicious chocolate oat zucchini cake is perfectly sweet, incredibly moist, and much healthier than a traditional chocolate cake. It is gluten-free, oil-free, and also rich in nutrients from the hidden vegetables and fruits. Coffee is a magic ingredient, which intensifies the chocolate flavor.

Ingredients

- ¾ cup (96ml) unsweetened soy milk
- 2 teaspoons apple cider vinegar
- ½ cup (125g) unsweetened applesauce
- ½ cup (62g) shredded zucchini
- 1 teaspoon vanilla extract
- ½ cup (65g) sugar
- ⅓ cup (35g) cocoa
- 1½ cups (190g) oat flour
- 1 tablespoon cornstarch
- 2 teaspoons instant coffee powder
- ½ teaspoon baking powder
- ½ teaspoon baking soda
- ¼ teaspoon salt

Variations

- Replace the zucchini with grated summer squash.
- Drizzle the cake with some drippy peanut butter or some melted dark chocolate to make it extra rich.
- Add blueberries or pitted cherries to the cake for extra fruity flavor.

Tools

- Grater
- Kitchen scale
- Large mixing bowl
- Measuring cups and spoons
- Parchment paper
- Round cake pan (9 inches)
- Spatula
- Toothpick
- Whisk

Instructions

1. Preheat the oven to 350°F (180°C) and line a round cake pan with parchment paper.
2. In a large mixing bowl, whisk the soy milk with the apple cider vinegar and let the mixture sit for 2 to 3 minutes, to form a vegan buttermilk.
3. Add the applesauce, shredded zucchini, vanilla, and sugar. Whisk everything together.
4. Add in the cocoa, oat flour, cornstarch, coffee, baking powder, baking soda, and salt. Gently stir with a spatula until all the ingredients are well-combined and a smooth batter forms.
5. Transfer the batter to the prepared baking pan and place it in the oven to bake for 25 to 30 minutes or until a toothpick inserted into the center comes out clean.
6. Let the cake cool to room temperature before slicing and serving.

Serving size: 1 slice
Calories per serving: 160
Macros: Carbohydrates: 32.1g; Fiber: 4g; Protein: 5g; Fat: 2g

FROZEN HONEY YOGURT BARK

PAREVE

Prep time: 10 minutes

Yield: 10 pieces

This frozen honey yogurt bark is the perfect light and refreshing dessert, especially for Rosh Hashanah. It comes together in no time and is a great option to make with your kids—they can choose their own toppings and have fun with adding things to the yogurt bark. It is also low in sugar and high in protein. Serve with napkins to clean up sticky hands!

Ingredients

- 2 cups (570g) plain Greek yogurt
- 3 tablespoons honey
- 2 teaspoons vanilla extract
- 2 tablespoons natural peanut butter
- 2 tablespoons strawberry jam, warmed
- 1 cup (125g) fresh strawberries, sliced
- ¼ cup (30g) pistachios, roughly chopped (or other nuts of choice)

Variations

- Use unsweetened soy or coconut yogurt to make the recipe dairy-free.
- Use any toppings of your choice: various nuts or dried fruit, jams, fresh fruit, nut butter, melted chocolate, mini marshmallows, or cupcake sprinkles for a birthday version.
- Add lemon zest, orange zest, peppermint extract, or almond extract to the yogurt for extra flavor.

Tools

- Kitchen scale
- Measuring cups and spoons
- Medium mixing bowl
- Parchment paper
- Rimmed baking sheet
- Spoon
- Toothpick

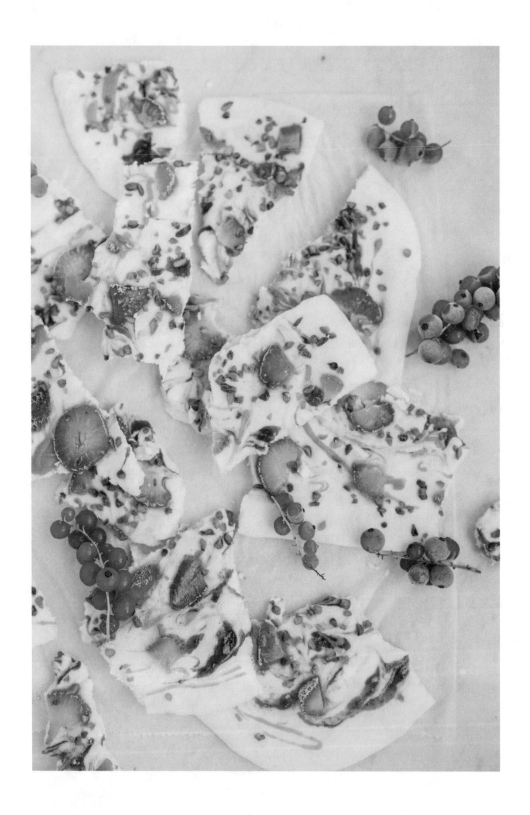

Instructions

1. In a medium mixing bowl, combine Greek yogurt, honey, and vanilla extract. Stir until smooth.

2. Line a rimmed baking sheet with a piece of parchment paper and spread the yogurt mixture on top.

3. Dollop the peanut butter and jam onto the yogurt and swirl using a toothpick.

4. Sprinkle on the toppings.

5. Transfer the yogurt bark to the freezer for 2 to 3 hours or until set. Slice or break into 10 pieces and serve immediately.

6. Keep leftovers in the freezer.

Serving size: 1 piece
Calories per serving: 110
Macros: Carbohydrates: 13.2g; Fiber: 1g; Protein: 8g; Fat: 3.1g

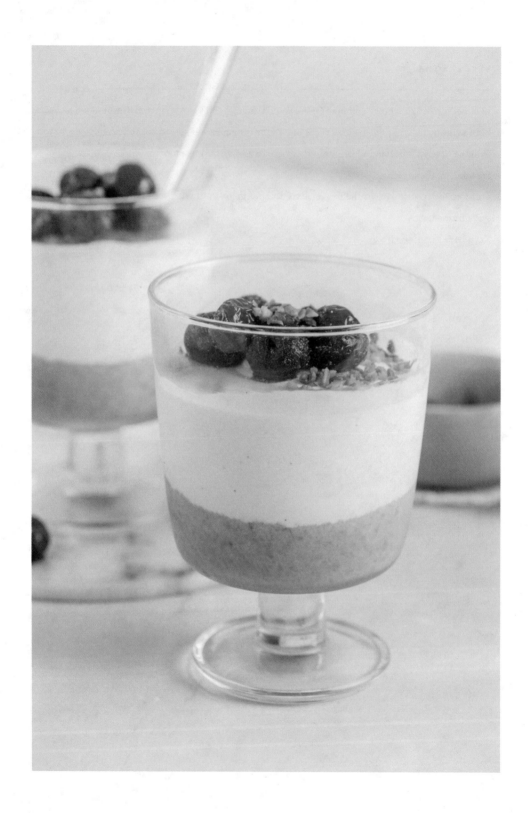

INDIVIDUAL CHERRY AND GRAHAM CRACKER "CHEESECAKE" PARFAIT

Prep time: 10 minutes | Chill time: 3 hours to overnight | Total time: 3 hours 10 minutes

Yield: 1 parfait

This recipe is inspired by one of the richest desserts: cheesecake. This healthy parfait is made with rich Greek yogurt and a touch of cream cheese, graham crackers, and fresh seasonal fruit. This gives you everything a cheesecake does, but with fewer calories, carbs, and lower fat content. Crunchy cookie bottom, creamy middle, and fresh and tangy fruit topping create a pleasurable dessert that can be enjoyed every day. Great for making in advance or scaling up for batch cooking.

Ingredients

- ¾ cup (170g) low-fat and high-protein Greek yogurt
- 1 teaspoon cream cheese
- ½ teaspoon guar gum powder
- ½ teaspoon stevia
- ½ teaspoon of vanilla extract
- 1 teaspoon lemon juice
- ½ teaspoon lemon zest
- 2 tablespoons crushed graham crumbs (1 graham cracker sheet, crushed)
- 5 fresh cherries, diced

Variations

- Use any fresh seasonal fruits for the topping.
- Instead of vanilla, use another flavor extract: almond, lemon, peppermint, coconut, and maple would all be delicious!
- Guar gum thickens the yogurt and cream cheese mixture. Leave it out for a thinner texture.

Tools

- Glass jars or ramekins
- Kitchen scale
- Measuring cups and spoons
- Medium mixing bowl
- Small bowl
- Whisk

Instructions

1. Place the yogurt, cream cheese, guar gum, stevia, vanilla, lemon juice, and lemon zest in a mixing bowl and whisk vigorously until smooth. If using guar gum, the mixture should thicken as you whisk.
2. Layer the ingredients in an 8-ounce jar. First, spread the graham cracker crumbs on the bottom. Then, add the cheesecake layer and push it down into the graham cracker crumbs. Finally, top with the diced cherries.
3. Chill for at least 1 hour. Keep refrigerated until serving.

Serving size: 1 parfait
Calories per serving: 212
Macros: Carbohydrates: 29g; Fiber: 1g; Protein: 18g; Fat: 5.9g

MARSHMALLOW, CHOCOLATE, AND GRAHAM CRACKER CREMBO BITES

PAREVE

Prep time: 20 minutes | Chill time: 1 to 2 hours | Total time: 2 hours 20 minutes

Yield: 12 crembo bites

These bite-sized cookies are a simplified version of the classic Israeli treat: a round cookie base with a chocolate-covered marshmallow on top. This five ingredient version delivers chocolate, nuts, marshmallow, and graham crackers all in one bite. These bite-sized individual desserts come together in less than twenty minutes.

Ingredients

- 10 ounces (285g) dark chocolate, chopped
- ½ cup (120g) natural peanut butter
- ⅓ cup (48g) almonds, roughly chopped
- ⅓ cup (36g) graham crackers, crumbled
- 1 cup (60g) mini marshmallows

Variations
- Replace the dark chocolate with white chocolate for a different flavor.
- Add dried fruits or coconut for extra flavor.

Tools

- Glass bowl (to sit over pan)
- Kitchen scale
- Measuring cups and spoons
- Medium mixing bowl
- Parchment paper
- Rimmed baking sheet
- Small pan

Instructions

1. Melt chocolate over a double boiler. Once melted, stir in the peanut butter and place in the refrigerator for 10 minutes.

2. Once the mixture is slightly cooled, stir in the almonds and graham crackers.

3. Finally, stir in the marshmallows at the end so they don't melt in the chocolate mixture.

4. Spoon the mixture onto a parchment-lined baking sheet. You should get around 12 crembo bites.

5. Place in the fridge to cool until set, around 1 to 2 hours.

Serving size: 1 crembo bite
Calories per serving: 225
Macros: Carbohydrates: 23g; Fiber: 3g; Protein: 5g; Fat: 16g

NO-BAKE WALNUT CINNAMON PROTEIN COOKIES

Prep time: 5 minutes | Chill time: 1 hour | Total time: 1 hour 5 minutes

Yield: 8 cookies

These no-bake, gluten-free protein cookies are nutty and smooth on the inside. They are easy to make, full of healthy ingredients, and irresistibly delicious. They are pretty too. Loaded with protein, fiber, and healthy fat—a perfect energizing and satisfying sweet treat any time of day.

Ingredients

- ¼ cup (60g) natural almond butter (preferably no added sugar or salt)
- 1 teaspoon vanilla extract
- ½ teaspoon ground cinnamon
- 2 teaspoons chia seeds
- 2 scoops vanilla protein powder
- 1 tablespoon coconut oil
- 8 walnut halves

Variations
- For a dairy-free option, use a plant-based protein powder.

Tools

- Airtight container
- Food processor
- Kitchen scale
- Measuring cups and spoons
- Parchment paper
- Plate

Instructions

1. Place almond butter, vanilla, cinnamon, chia seeds, protein powder, and coconut oil in a food processor. Pulse until the mixture forms a thick paste, then stop immediately. Over-processing will cause the mixture to become too sticky.

2. Form the dough into 8 equal balls using slightly damp hands.

3. Place the balls on a plate lined with baking parchment, and flatten slightly. Press a walnut half into the top of each.

4. Transfer the protein cookies to the fridge to firm up for at least 1 hour. Once firm, transfer to an airtight container and store in the fridge for up to 1 week.

Serving size: 1 cookie
Calories: 113
Macros: Carbohydrates: 5.7g; Fiber: 3g; Protein: 9.5g; Fat: 7.6g

OATMEAL CHOCOLATE CHIP COOKIES

PAREVE

Prep time: 10 minutes | Cook time: 15 minutes | Total time: 25 minutes

Yield: 24 cookies

These mini oatmeal chocolate chip cookies are soft, moist, delicious, and so healthy that you can even eat them for breakfast. This is a cookie recipe that comes together in just 10 minutes, that the whole family will love, and that is packed with fiber and nutrients from the fruit, oats, flax, and nut butter.

Ingredients

- 1 overripe banana
- 1 tablespoon ground flax
- 2 tablespoons water
- 1 tablespoon honey or agave
- 1 tablespoon coconut oil, liquid form
- ¼ cup hazelnut butter (or any nut or seed butter of choice)
- 1 teaspoon vanilla extract
- 1 cup rolled oats
- ½ teaspoon baking powder
- ½ cup dark chocolate chips

Variations

- Replace the banana with canned pumpkin puree or applesauce for a different flavor.
- Switch out the chocolate chips for raisins or dried cranberries for a fruity twist.
- Use any nut butter—peanut butter and almond butter work well.
- Instead of coconut oil, use vegan butter spread or real butter.
- Make a double batch and freeze some.

Tools

- Fork
- Kitchen scale
- Large mixing bowl
- Measuring cups and spoons
- Parchment paper
- Rimmed baking sheet
- Whisk

Instructions

1. Preheat the oven to 375°F (190°C) and line a rimmed baking sheet with a piece of parchment paper.

2. In a large mixing bowl, mash the banana with a fork until smooth.

3. Add in the ground flax, water, honey, coconut oil, hazelnut butter, and vanilla; whisk until smooth and creamy.

4. Add in the oats, baking powder, and chocolate chips; mix until combined. The mixture will be loose—this is fine.

5. Drop tablespoon-sized scoops of the dough onto the prepared baking sheet. Lightly press into a circle shape—the cookies won't spread and will hold their shape while baking. You should get around 10 medium-sized cookies.

6. Place in the oven to bake until golden brown and crispy around the edges, around 12 to 15 minutes. Leave to cool slightly before serving.

Serving size: 1 cookie
Calories per serving: 62
Macros: Carbohydrates: 6.8g; Fiber: 0.8g; Protein: 1.1g; Fat: 3.5g

RAW BROWNIE BITES

PAREVE

Prep time: 10 minutes

Yield: 30 bites (1 tablespoon each)

These raw brownie bites are a rich treat to satisfy your daily chocolate craving. They are made from black beans, giving them a smooth texture and a protein and fiber boost. I learned to love using beans in sweet desserts and snacks while living in Asia, where it is common practice. They taste just like classic brownies!

Ingredients

- ½ cup (50g) + 2 tablespoons unsweetened cocoa
- 1 cup (180–200g) cooked black beans, drained and rinsed
- ½ cup (120g) peanut butter (or almond butter)
- ¼ cup (85g) honey or maple syrup
- ½ cup (45g) rolled oats
- 1 teaspoon vanilla
- 3 tablespoons oat milk
- Pinch of salt

Variations
- Replace the oats with quinoa flakes to make gluten-free and/or kosher for Passover.
- Replace the black beans with white beans.

- To serve for a special occasion, place a piece of chocolate or one almond into each bite.

Tools

- Food processor
- Kitchen scale
- Measuring cups and spoons
- Rubber spatula

Instructions

1. Pulse cocoa, black beans, peanut butter, honey, oats, vanilla, oat milk, and salt in a food processor until thoroughly combined and the batter starts to clump together and the oats disappear. This takes longer than you might think.

2. Using a tablespoon as a measuring guide, make 30 equal balls.

3. Eat immediately or store in an airtight container and place in the refrigerator.

Serving size: 1 brownie bite
Calories per serving: 45
Macros: Carbohydrates: 5.3g; Fiber: 1g; Protein: 1.5g; Fat: 2.5g

SOUR CREAM COFFEE CAKE
WITH A CINNAMON SWIRL

Prep time: 10 minutes | Cook time: 40 minutes | Total time: 50 minutes

Yield: 16 servings

A healthier take on the classic coffee cake, this sour cream coffee cake with a cinnamon swirl is rich, moist, perfectly spiced, and very easy to prepare. It's perfect to serve for an afternoon treat with a cup of coffee or tea.

Ingredients

- 2 cups (250g) all-purpose flour
- 1 teaspoon baking powder
- 1 teaspoon baking soda
- ¼ teaspoon salt
- ¼ cup (60ml) coconut oil, at room temperature (not melted)
- ¾ cup (150g) sugar
- ¼ cup (62g) unsweetened applesauce
- 2 eggs
- 1 cup (245g) sour cream
- 1 tablespoon vanilla extract
- ¼ cup (50g) light brown sugar
- 1 tablespoon ground cinnamon

Variations

- Replace the sour cream with Greek yogurt to reduce the fat content.
- Replace the coconut oil with applesauce for an oil-free cake.
- Skip the cinnamon swirl and use jam instead.

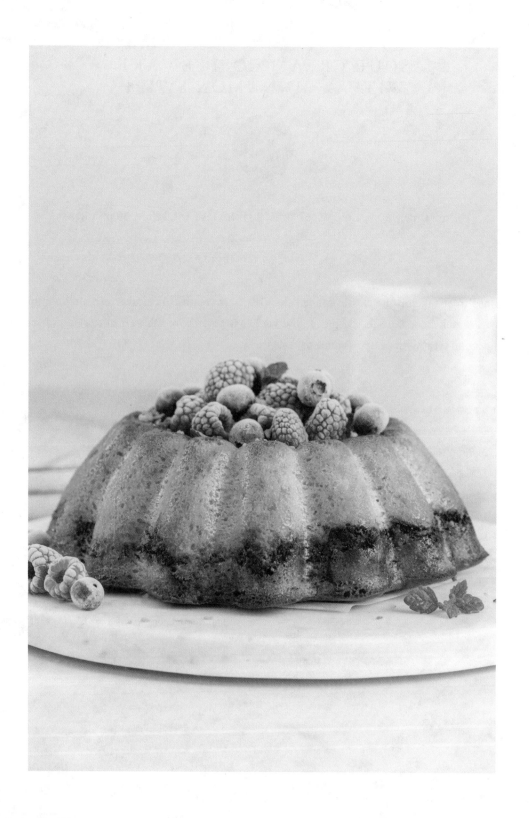

Tools

- Baking pan (9 x 13-inch) or Bundt cake pan
- Kitchen scale
- Large mixing bowl
- Measuring cups and spoons
- Medium mixing bowl
- Parchment paper
- Small mixing bowl
- Toothpick
- Whisk

Instructions

1. Preheat the oven to 350°F (180°C) and line a 9 x 13-inch baking pan with a piece of parchment paper.

2. In a medium mixing bowl, whisk together the flour, baking powder, baking soda, and salt. Set aside.

3. In a large mixing bowl, combine the coconut oil and sugar; whisk until light and fluffy, for at least 2 to 3 minutes.

4. Add in the applesauce, eggs, sour cream, and vanilla. Continue whisking until smoothly combined.

5. Gradually add the dry ingredients into the wet, folding to combine.

6. In a small mixing bowl, mix together the brown sugar and cinnamon.

7. Spread ⅔ of the coffee cake batter on the bottom of your prepared baking pan and sprinkle the cinnamon sugar mixture on top. Add the remaining batter and lightly swirl with a toothpick or a wooden skewer.

8. Bake until a toothpick inserted into the center comes out clean, around 35 to 40 minutes.

9. Leave to cool completely before slicing and serving.

Serving size: 1 slice
Calories per serving: 170
Macros: Carbohydrates: 25.5g; Fiber: 0.5g; Protein: 2.7g; Fat: 6.7g

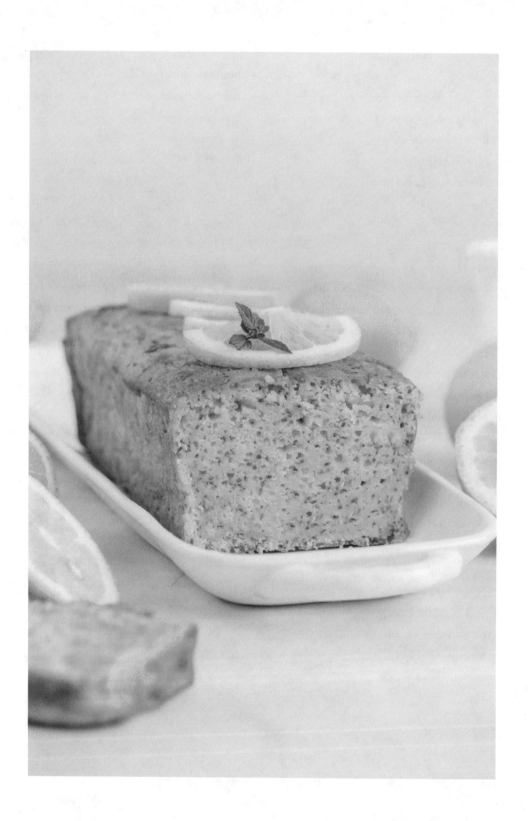

SPELT LEMON POPPY SEED LOAF CAKE

PAREVE

Prep time: 10 minutes | Cook time: 1 hour | Total time: 1 hour 10 minutes

Yield: 10 servings

This moist, golden, and lightly sweet spelt lemon poppy seed loaf cake is like sunshine on a plate. It has a light and tender crumb, yet it is easier to digest thanks to the spelt flour. The lovely golden color comes from the ground turmeric—this is a secret tip that will give all your cakes a wonderful yellow color.

Ingredients

- ½ cup (100g) white sugar
- 2 cups (250g) spelt flour
- 2 tablespoons poppy seeds
- 1 teaspoon baking powder
- ½ teaspoon baking soda
- ½ teaspoon ground turmeric
- 1 teaspoon lemon zest
- 1 cup (240ml) unsweetened soy milk
- ½ cup (123g) vegan soy or coconut yogurt (can be replaced with Greek yogurt if not dairy-free)
- 2 tablespoons melted coconut oil or vegetable oil
- Juice of 3 medium lemons
- 2 teaspoons vanilla extract

Variations

- Replace the lemon zest and juice with orange zest and juice for a flavor variation.
- Bake as muffins or a Bundt cake—just adjust the baking time as needed.
- Serve with a cream cheese glaze or with some lemon curd for extra deliciousness.

Tools

- Citrus juicer
- Kitchen scale
- Large mixing bowl
- Loaf pan
- Measuring cups and spoons
- Parchment paper
- Spatula
- Whisk
- Wooden spoon

Instructions

1. Preheat the oven to 375°F (190°C) and line a loaf pan with a piece of parchment paper, leaving a bit of overhang on the sides for easy removal.

2. In a large mixing bowl, combine sugar, flour, poppy seeds, baking powder, baking soda, turmeric, and lemon zest. Whisk until combined.

3. Add in the soy milk, yogurt, coconut oil, lemon juice, and vanilla. Gently mix until all the ingredients are combined and the batter is mostly smooth—a few lumps are fine. Do not overmix or the cake might turn out tough.

4. Pour the batter into the prepared loaf pan and place in the oven to bake until the cake is golden brown and a toothpick inserted into the center comes out clean, around 50 to 60 minutes.

5. Leave the cake to cool completely at room temperature before slicing and serving.

Serving size: 1 slice
Calories per serving: 180
Macros: Carbohydrates: 32.3g; Fiber: 4g; Protein: 5.5g; Fat: 4.5g

TAHINI MAPLE SESAME COOKIES

PAREVE

Prep time: 15 minutes + 10 minutes for the dough to rest | Cook time:
10 to 12 minutes | Total time: 37 minutes

Yield: 20 cookies

These gluten-free tahini cookies are my personal favorite: a special buttery, nutty taste with caramel sweetness. When you make them, make sure to use smooth, runny tahini. These cookies use a vegan baking trick of combining apple cider vinegar and baking soda to help the dough rise, resulting in a light cookie which is soft on the inside and crunchy on the outside.

Ingredients

- 1½ cups (145g) almond flour
- ½ cup (120g) tahini
- ¼ cup (70g) maple syrup
- 1 teaspoon vanilla extract
- 1 teaspoon apple cider vinegar
- ¾ teaspoon baking soda
- Pinch of sea salt (if needed)
- 1 to 2 tablespoons unsweetened plant-based milk (if needed)
- ¼ cup (35g) toasted sesame seeds

Variations
- Add chopped crystalized ginger.
- Use runny honey instead of maple syrup.
- Add ¼ cup of dark chocolate chips and skip the sesame seeds.
- Use almond extract instead of vanilla extract.

Tools

- Kitchen scale
- Large mixing bowl
- Measuring cups and spoons
- Parchment paper
- Rimmed baking sheet
- Small plate
- Spatula

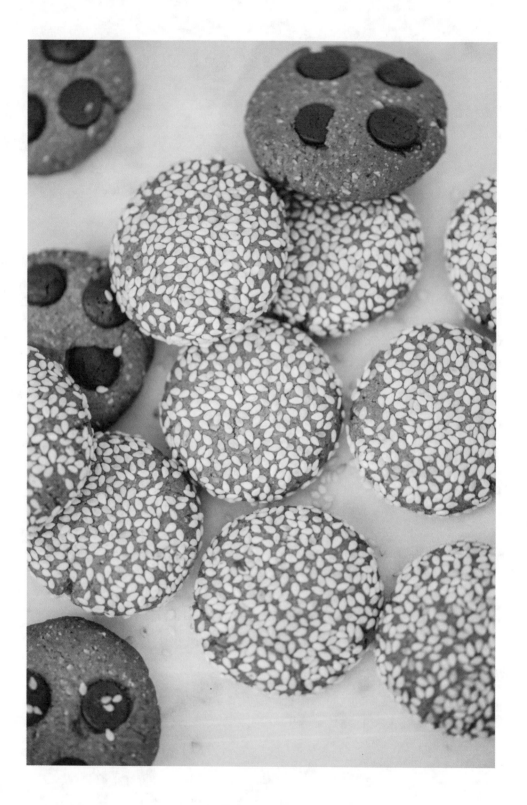

Instructions

1. Line a baking sheet with parchment paper.

2. Add almond flour, tahini, maple syrup, vanilla, apple cider vinegar, and baking soda to a mixing bowl. Using a spatula, mix until a moldable dough forms.

3. If the dough is too dry to roll into balls (for example, because your tahini was more solid than runny), add 1 to 2 tablespoons of plant-based milk and mix again. Keep mixing until you get a dough that can be easily shaped into cookies.

4. Taste the dough and add salt if needed. (Some tahinis have a naturally salty taste so this step depends on preference).

5. Turn on the oven to 350°F (180°C). Let the dough rest in the fridge for 10 minutes while the oven warms up.

6. Place the toasted sesame seeds on a small plate.

7. Form the dough into 20 balls, using a tablespoon as a guide.

8. Carefully roll each ball in the sesame seeds to coat, and place on the baking sheet.

9. Use your hands to gently flatten each ball into a cookie shape.

10. Bake cookies for about 10 to 12 minutes until golden brown around the edges. Check from time to time to avoid overbaking.

11. Remove from the oven and allow to cool and firm for at least 10 minutes before serving.

12. Store in an airtight container in the refrigerator for up to 7 days.

Serving size: 1 cookie
Calories per serving: 70
Macros: Carbohydrates: 4.8g; Fiber: 1g; Protein: 1.8g; Fat: 5.3g

APPENDICES

APPENDIX A

CALCULATE YOUR MACROS WORKSHEET

Here is a simple worksheet to calculate your ideal calorie intake and macronutrient targets, that you can tweak to:

- Maintain your body weight
- Increase your body weight
- Decrease your body weight

Remember, the target number this sheet gives you will only be a guide. Expect to do a little trial, error, and tweaking to find the macros balance that works best for you.

HOW TO CALCULATE YOUR DAILY CALORIE REQUIREMENTS

Find your Total Daily Energy Expenditure (TDEE) by using an online calculator. To find this online, simply google "Mifflin St. Jeor Calculator." You will be able to input age, height, current weight, and activity level and get your daily calorie requirements.

This simple method will give you an approximate range of how many calories you need every day in order to maintain your weight. The result will not be 100 percent accurate because our individual bodies are not generic machines. We all have different metabolisms, genetics, activity levels, etc. Use this number as a guide for how many calories you need to consume in order to maintain your current weight, and tweak it as needed.

If your body weight range falls in the overweight or obese categories, according to the body mass index (BMI) standards for your biological sex, use the highest normal weight number/lowest overweight number for your height and age in the BMI standards as your "current weight" in the above equation.

NEXT STEPS

1.   Use the estimated calorie value and consume around this number of calories every day for a week.
2.   During this time, weigh yourself every morning (naked and on an empty stomach) and monitor weight changes for one week.
3.   If your weight doesn't change, this number is your "maintenance calories number": the number of calories you need to consume daily to maintain your weight.
4.   If you lose weight, then your maintenance calories number is higher.
5.   If you gain weight, then your maintenance calories number is lower.

HOW TO CREATE THE OPTIMAL CALORIE DEFICIT OR SURPLUS TO LOSE OR GAIN WEIGHT

Once you have your Daily Calorie Requirements number (TDEE), you can subtract or add calories depending on if you want to lose or gain weight. If you want to lose weight you need to be in a calorie deficit (to eat fewer calories than your body needs to maintain your weight). If you want to gain weight, you will have to be in a calorie surplus (to eat more calories than you need to maintain your weight).

To decrease your body weight: TDEE Calorie Number _____ - 250 to 500 calories = _____ Deficit calorie number

To increase your body weight: TDEE Calorie Number _____ + 300 calories = _____ = Surplus calorie number

FILL IN THE BLANKS TO CALCULATE YOUR DAILY MACRONUTRIENT TARGETS IN GRAMS AND CALORIES

These calculations are less complicated than they seem, so go step-by-step.

CALORIES PER GRAM OF MACRONUTRIENT

- 1 gram of protein = 4 calories
- 1 gram of carbohydrate = 4 calories
- 1 gram of fat = 9 calories

CALCULATE PROTEIN NEEDS FIRST

The optimal protein intake is about 1.2–2.4 g/kg of body weight (0.5–1.10 g/lb) per day, but the range may vary according to your age and activity level.

- If you are overweight (according to the BMI), use your target body weight rather than your current body weight; when it comes to protein needs, aim for 1.2–1.5 g/kg (0.5–0.7 g/lb)
- If you are lean (<10% body fat for males and <20% body fat for females), aim for 1g protein per pound of body weight; aim for 1.6–2.4 g/kg (0.7–1.10 g/lb)
- If you are eating in a calorie deficit to lose body fat, aim for 1.6–2.4 g/kg (0.7–1.10 g/lb)

PROTEIN GRAMS AND CALORIES PER DAY

Total body weight (lbs) _____ × 0.8 = Grams of protein per day _____

Grams of protein _____ × 4 calories per gram = _____ Protein calories per day

FAT GRAMS AND CALORIES PER DAY

Total body weight (lbs) _____ × 0.25-0.45 = Grams of fat per day _____

Grams of fat _____ × 9 calories per gram = _____ Calories from fat

CARBOHYDRATE GRAMS AND CALORIES PER DAY

Total calories per day _____ - Protein calories per day _____ - Fat calories
per day = _____ Carbohydrate calories per day

Calories coming from carbohydrates per day _____ ÷ 4 = _____
Carbohydrates grams per day

Total Calories	Protein Grams	Fat Grams	Carbohydrate Grams

WHAT'S NEXT

Take the above calorie and macronutrient goals and put them into MyFitnessPal (see tracking step-by-step worksheet).

Please note: If you are using macros to lose body fat, it is recommended to stay in a calorie deficit for 12 to 16 weeks, or until you reach your goal weight. Staying in a calorie deficit beyond this timeframe is not helpful for your body or mind.

If you are trying to lose a large amount of body fat, most people have better results when they do so over a long period of time going through a few cycles of a calorie deficit of 12 to 16 weeks followed by maintenance rather than staying in a calorie deficit for an extended period of time.

FOR FUTURE REFERENCE

If you are using macros to lose body fat, "reverse dieting" is an approach that can be useful when moving from calorie deficit back to maintenance calories. Please see the explanation of reverse dieting on page 186.

APPENDIX B

TRACKING MACROS, STEP-BY-STEP

A central pillar of this eating framework is accurately tracking the food you eat, every day, for a period of time (remember that it is not forever). The goal of tracking is to help you understand how many calories you consume, how much of each macronutrient (carbohydrate, protein, and fat) you are eating, and what a balanced portion size looks like for you. The skill of appropriate portion sizing is important for lifelong weight management.

HOW A FOOD JOURNAL CAN SUPPORT YOU

Tracking is not about "getting in trouble" for food choices. It is a neutral tool to capture data to help you with lifelong weight management and overall health.

Noting the amount of energy (calories) consumed daily is essential because you maintain, lose, or gain weight depending on it.

When you want to lose weight, you need to create a calorie deficit, where you use more calories than you eat. To create a calorie surplus in order to gain weight, you need to eat more calories than you use.

When we estimate (rather than calculate) the number of calories we eat, we will usually end up off the mark. We might forget about things we eat unconsciously while doing other tasks, have a skewed sense of portions, or not recognize that we have eaten an inadequate amount of food. Using a food diary–type app that tracks the amount of food consumed proves much more effective. With its help, you can measure the calories consumed more accurately, giving you a clear picture of what you eat and how it measures up against your calorie and macronutrient target numbers.

MYFITNESSPAL EXPLAINED

Using an app to track your macros is a time- and labor-saving option. There are lots of food diary apps to choose from, so choose the one that suits you. I recommend My-FitnessPal because this is what I have personally used for tracking, and I found it very user-friendly. When I first started tracking, I felt overwhelmed and watched YouTube videos and read blogs about how to use MyFitnessPal for tracking. Hopefully the following summary will save you time and give you all the information you need to be able to get started right away!

MyFitnessPal is a diary-type application that aims to help people record the food that they eat. The idea is that it is possible to manage something you can measure. Please note that the below directions are from the 2022 app and MyFitnessPal might change. Regardless, the details below will give you a sense about how to track.

MyFitnessPal contains a large database of foods, along with their nutritional information. Simply enter what you eat and how much in the diary, and the app will automatically calculate your daily calorie intake. It will also display a ratio of how many carbs, fats, and proteins you have consumed. This makes it simple for you to review if you are on track to meeting your daily calorie and nutrient goals.

Immediately after installation and launch, MyFitnessPal puts the user through a short set of questions about their physical characteristics (age, height, weight, regular physical activity), as well as their goal—if they want to maintain, lose, or gain weight. This app processes this data and calculates a suggested daily calorie target that the user should try to meet, with options to select for faster or slower results. A daily maximum calorie target is set, and the app will use this as a base for providing data about your progress every day.

For each day, MyFitnessPal allows the entry of data on drinking water, food consumed (breakfast, lunch, dinner, snacks between meals), physical activity, and changes in body weight. Of these, only food consumption data is "required"—if the user forgets to provide data for a particular meal of the day, they will receive a few discreet reminder notifications to do so.

STEP ONE: CREATE THE ACCOUNT

- Download the app
- Click on "sign up now"
- Follow the on-screen instructions to get started

STEP TWO: SET YOUR CALORIES

Establish the target for daily calorie intake. This can be automatically done after entering your details (current weight, age, height, sex, activity level, and goals). You can also adjust the number of calories according to your preference.

STEP 3: SET YOUR MARCOS TARGET NUMBER

You need to fix the daily ratio for each macronutrient (proteins, carbohydrates, and fats). To do this, click on "Goals," where you'll see your "Daily Nutrition Goals," and you can either use the recommended ratio, which is 50 percent carbohydrates, 20 percent protein, and 30 percent fat, or you can adjust it as you wish. After this, the app will calculate how many grams of each macronutrient you should eat daily.

STEP 4: PLAN AND TRACK YOUR FOOD

Once you've set your macros, it's time to record everything you eat in the app. You can do this in three ways:

1. Food scanning

MyFitnessPal has a code scanner function which can be used to easily pull up nutritional data on prepackaged food and ingredients. Simply scan the barcode like this:

1. Open the app and click on the blue "Add" button at the bottom of the screen.
2. Press the orange "food" button.
3. Choose the meal you want to record (breakfast, lunch, dinner, or snack).
4. Tap the barcode symbol at the top right of the screen.
5. Scan the food barcode.
6. Enter the portion size if necessary.

2. Search and add

To record foods without a barcode, such as fruits, vegetables, meats, etc.:

1. Open MyFitnessPal and press the blue "Add" button at the bottom of the screen.
2. Press the orange "food" button.
3. Choose the meal you want to record (breakfast, lunch, dinner, or snack).
4. Click the "search for food" tab and enter the name of the food you are looking for.
5. Do not rush to choose the first result that appears; scroll through the list to find the most precise option.
6. Choose the food and add the quantity.
7. Press "enter."

After using MyFitnessPal for a while, a list of recently added foods is created. This cuts down the time you spend recording items that you eat regularly.

3. Quick Add

Sometimes you might know the total calorie content of a dish, but not its specific ingredients. This is useful when eating at restaurants where the calories are displayed on the menu.

1. Open MyFitnessPal and press the blue "Add" button at the bottom of the screen.
2. Press the orange "food" button.
3. Choose the meal you want to record (breakfast, lunch, dinner, or snack).
4. Go to the bottom of the page and select "quick add."
5. You can enter the number of calories you eat. If you have a premium account, you can also add the amount of protein, carbohydrates, and fats.

As you enter meals and snacks into your food diary, MyFitnessPal will total how many grams of carbohydrates, fat, and protein you've eaten.

STEP FIVE: REPEAT AND REFINE

A food journal helps you eat more responsibly. When you decide to eat healthier, keeping a food diary brings you closer to your goal. By noting the food you eat, you become more aware of how much you eat, what you eat, and most importantly, why. The food diary helps you identify and reduce episodes of compulsive eating due to boredom or emotions.

APPENDIX C

TRACKING PRO-TIPS

Here is a list of tracking best practices to make the act of meeting calorie and macronutrient goals more efficient and enjoyable for you. You might already be doing some of these naturally!

FOOD SCALE

To accurately track food intake, a food scale is essential. People tend to underestimate how much they are eating, and rely on sight alone to measure portions of food. The best way to determine the size of a meal at home is by using a kitchen scale. Remember, it's not forever! Using a food scale for a period of time allows you to familiarize yourself with accurate portion sizes. After a while, you won't need to weigh food because eating the right portion sizes will become a habit. This is an essential part of the foundations of sustainable weight management.

CALORIES AND PROTEIN GOALS FIRST

When you first get started, meeting calories plus all three macronutrient goals can feel overwhelming. First, focus on meeting your calorie and protein goal and let your carbohydrate and fat numbers vary.

TRACK PLANNED FOOD IN THE MORNING BEFORE YOUR DAYS START

Planning meals in the morning helps! Start with either your favorite meal of the day or the meal you know. For example, if you eat the same breakfast every day, log that first and fill your day in around it.

With time, both the planning and the execution of eating macros-balanced meals tend to get easier. In the beginning, you will probably find the way you plan and eat feels quite structured. During this phase, you build your repertoire of recipes and favorite food combinations and repeat those often. After time, planning and execution—including allowing for special occasions and meals—becomes second nature.

Planning also prevents you from reaching dinnertime with 5 grams of carbs and 100 grams of protein left in your daily targets. This can lead to some unbalanced and unusual meal combinations, which is counterintuitive to the goal of macros: eating everything for physical and emotional balance.

TRACK EMOTIONAL MUST-HAVE DAILY FOODS FIRST

We all have foods that we are emotionally attached to and miss when we don't include them in our diet. We should eat all foods in moderation so that we do not dip into feelings of food deprivation. Track the foods you love first and build your daily meal plan around them.

- If you need to have a piece of dark chocolate every day, track it!
- If you want to enjoy challah bread every Shabbat dinner, track it!

INDIVIDUAL-SIZED SWEET AND SAVORY TREATS

1. Remember that no food is forbidden or banned! With that being said, it is also true that it is easy to overindulge in sweet and savory treats. One way to enjoy a moderate amount of treats every day is to buy and consume individual-sized portions of them. For example, rather than buying a family-sized bag of your favorite potato chips, buy individually portioned sized bags. Instead of buying your favorite chocolate bar, buy individual chocolate pieces, etc.

REPEAT AND REFINE RECIPES
AND INGREDIENT LISTS

Let's be honest, it takes time to find and cook new recipes three times a day! It's better to make things easy for yourself by eating the same group of recipes every day, or repeating meals and ingredients throughout the week. This simple approach may help you lose weight or stick with your diet, especially at the beginning. As you get more used to this eating pattern, you can vary things without feeling overwhelmed. A simple tip is to make your dinner large enough to have leftovers the next day for lunch. Meal prepping can be time consuming, and this is an easy way to ensure you have food made the next day.

MOVE CALORIES TO DIFFERENT DAYS

One way to think about calories is as a weekly budget. In this way, it is possible to shift calories from one meal or one day to another, to accommodate the flexibility for normal daily life as well as for special occasions.

FOR EXAMPLE:

- You know you are going to a restaurant for dinner on Saturday and you want to enjoy the full meal with dessert. So, you might have a lighter lunch that day, or even reduce your calorie intake slightly for the 2 preceding days.
- You have a birthday party to attend and you will enjoy a piece of cake. So you decide to keep your carbohydrates and fats lower at meals throughout that day.
- You enjoy a croissant and cappuccino for breakfast, which you balance with a protein-rich lunch and dinner.

This is not the concept of a "cheat meal" and should not be taken to the extreme. These calorie *micro* adjustments are meant to give you food flexibility and allow you to enjoy special foods from time to time.

If you feel moving calories around triggers disordered eating thoughts or behaviors, then it's best to not use it as a tool.

KEEP YOURSELF HYDRATED (WITH WATER)

Drinking enough water each day is crucial for body functioning and mood stability. Most of us could drink more water than we currently do. Thirst signals can also be confused with hunger signals. By ensuring you are taking in plenty of water (and other fluids), you can be free to interpret hunger signals as what they are: signs you need to eat!

If it's hard for you to drink plain water, try adding fresh lemon juice, slices of cucumber and fresh mint sprigs, or brewing herbal teas to enjoy hot, lukewarm, or cold.

Another hydration tip: In the morning, fill jars, glasses, or bottles with your daily water intake goal—aim for 2 to 3 liters of water. Leave them in plain sight or in the refrigerator, and by the end of the day you will know for sure whether you have hydrated yourself enough that day.

DRINKING CALORIES

As a general rule, it's best not to drink calories, and to be mindful of consumption of high-sugar drinks including fruit juices and milky coffee drinks, hot chocolate, etc. Many of these drinks are calorie-rich but offer little to no nutritional value. It's more satisfying to eat calories and meet your daily energy needs from more nutritious foods such as vegetables, legumes, fruits, nuts, seeds, whole grains, and lean meats.

ACCURACY WHEN TRACKING FOOD

When you track food, you are trying to get an accurate picture of the calories and macronutrients you consume. When you start tracking on MyFitnessPal, you will see there are different nutrition values for similar food items. When eating packaged or canned food, scan the barcode. When eating fresh vegetables, meats, fish, or dairy, weigh it! This way, you will be sure that your tracking process is more accurate.

ENJOYING RESTAURANTS WHILE TRACKING

Eating out is part of life, and it is possible to enjoy eating in restaurants while tracking.

- Stick with simple food combinations and pay attention to the serving size mentioned on the menu.
- Check out the menu in advance. Some restaurant chains are already on MyFitnessPal, and therefore meals from their menus are already listed. Otherwise, you can track similar items that you think have an approximate equivalent nutritional value to the dishes you choose.
- Understand this is not the most accurate way to track. If you want to track precisely in order to reach specific health goals, be mindful about how often you eat in restaurants versus preparing meals at home.

CALORIES ARE NOT ALL NUTRITIONALLY EQUAL

When tracking calories and macros, you should also consider the actual quality of the food. It is possible to meet your daily calorie intake goal of 2,000 kcals without nourishing yourself. For example, if you primarily base your plate on calorie-dense foods like chocolate, french fries, nuts, and fast foods, your calorie budget will be exhausted without giving you enough vitamins, minerals, protein, and fiber.

A better approach is to focus on nutrient-dense foods first. Fill your plate with vegetables, whole grains, low-fat milk products, fish, lean meats, eggs, beans, nuts, and fresh fruits. Then fill in the gaps with calorie-rich foods, safe in the knowledge that you've already fueled your body with plenty of vitamins, minerals, complex carbohydrates, lean protein, and healthy fats.

Most people find that they feel at their physical and mental/emotional best spending 80 to 90 percent of their daily calories on minimally processed whole foods like fruits, vegetables, high-quality proteins, nuts, seeds, and starches and whole grains. The remaining 10 to 20 percent of the daily calorie budget can be spent on fun foods and treats, however you define them.

APPENDIX D

FOUR PHASES OF MACROS TRACKING

Macros tracking has four distinct phases that are used to achieve specific goals.

BULKING

WHAT IS IT?

This phase describes eating a caloric surplus with the aim of causing weight gain, and using particular physical activities to convert this gain to muscle mass.

ANYTHING ELSE TO KNOW?

Many things, including age, hormones, and genetic factors, influence how a person gains muscle mass. A macros coach can help make sure bulking results in increased muscle, not just weight gain.

CUTTING

WHAT IS IT?

Eating a caloric deficit with the aim of causing fat loss. This may seem like regular dieting. However, within the macros dietary pattern calorie deficits are usually small and go along with tweaking macronutrient ratios to attain sustainable weight loss goals.

ANYTHING ELSE TO KNOW?

Again, age, hormones, genetic factors, and various other factors influence how a person loses body fat. Cutting is not about getting calories to the lowest possible number in an attempt to see rapid weight loss. Nor is it about yo-yoing between restriction and overconsumption. Rather, the aim is to find a reasonable calorie deficit that you can follow and manage for 8 to 12 weeks to achieve or get closer to your goals.

MAINTENANCE

WHAT IS IT?

People eat in a calorie deficit (cut) or calorie surplus (bulk) for a limited amount of time only. For the majority of the time, people will be in the maintenance phase—consuming the calorie number and macronutrient ratio which maintains their body weight. Some people enter maintenance when they reach their goals and some people (especially those aiming to lose or gain a larger quantity of weight) will alternate from maintenance to cut/bulk phase several times until they reach their goals.

ANYTHING ELSE TO KNOW?

The transition from a calorie deficit or surplus to maintenance is called "reverse dieting."

REVERSE DIETING

WHAT IS IT?

Gradually increasing calorie intake (over a period of weeks or months) after eating in a calorie deficit, in order to stimulate the metabolism so the body burns more calories throughout the day.

ANYTHING ELSE TO KNOW?

Reverse dieting is a time-limited phase, implemented to avoid regaining weight when coming out of a period of eating in a calorie deficit.

When we feed the body less than it needs in order to lose weight, the metabolism slows down to conserve energy. Slowly increasing calorie intake gives the metabolism the signal to speed back up and the time to adjust to using more calories again.

Skipping the reverse dieting phase and returning to eating a higher number of calories right away causes weight gain, which in turn often prompts a return to eating in deficit again. This sudden stop-start approach to calorie intake is called yo-yo dieting, and causes the familiar cycle of weight gain and loss.

HOW TO IMPLEMENT REVERSE DIETING

Remember that a person should only stay in a calorie deficit for a limited period of time. When you reach your goal weight, or get closer to it, it's time to stop eating in a calorie deficit.

WHAT TO DO

- Increase calorie intake gradually—start by increasing daily intake by 50 to 100 calories and stick to this for two to three weeks.
- Continue to increase calorie intake by increments, allowing the body two to three weeks to adjust each time. Repeat until you reach the desired number of calories.

THINGS TO NOTICE

- Monitor average weight at the end of each week: calculate the average using daily weight readings taken first thing every morning. As daily weight tends to fluctuate, using a weekly average gives a more accurate overall view. Note: some weight gain is normal during a reverse diet, and should slow down as the metabolism adapts to the increase. If weight increases rapidly or significantly, wait another week or two before making another increase.

- Notice bodily responses to the increase in calories: energy levels, hunger, and sleep. You may notice increases in energy, physical endurance (such as gym performance), hunger cues, and quality of sleep.
- Prioritize movement during the reverse dieting phase. Move your body three to five days per week and stay active outside of focused "exercise" periods—tracking steps is a great way to do this.
- Keep tracking your food intake.

REMEMBER

The reverse dieting phase is about giving your body more calories and not about returning to unhealthy eating habits. Lifelong weight management is about eating a balanced diet and enjoying regular movement.

APPENDIX E

WAYS TO MEASURE PROGRESS

Consistently meeting macros goals leads to measurable progress in the following three areas:

- Physique: form, size, and development of your body
- Internal body functioning
- Relationship with food

MEASURING PROGRESS WITH YOUR PHYSIQUE: FORM, SIZE, AND DEVELOPMENT OF YOUR BODY

- **Body weight:** Weighing yourself every day allows you to understand how your body weight varies throughout the month (especially for women) and learn how to accept these natural body weight variations. The number on the scale is neutral data about your body; it does not reflect your personal value.
- Expect daily weight fluctuations on the scale. The body retains different amounts of water depending on food intake and activity level. Look for an overall trend across weeks and months to gauge progress.
- **Weekly measurements:** Measuring change in inches or centimeters provides information about the size and form of your body that may not be reflected in your weight. Measure around the bust, waist, buttocks, and the thickness of the thigh in the most prominent area. For information about more subtle changes, measure the most voluminous part of the biceps and calves.
- **Photographs:** Taking pictures of yourself once a week or every month can track changes in your physical appearance and complexion. Wear the same clothes,

take the pictures at the same time in the same place and stand with good posture against a clean wall to take pictures from the front, side, and back.

MEASURING PROGRESS WITH YOUR INTERNAL BODY FUNCTIONING

- **Measure physical strength and endurance:** Monitoring your physical strength and endurance gives you information about your muscle mass and body composition.
- Do a fitness test (how many push-ups, burpees, and squats you manage to do, for example).
- Measure how fast or how long you are able to run or walk over a specific distance.
- Notice changes in how you feel after doing regular tasks: is climbing the stairs different? Is a route you often walk getting easier?
- **Sleep, hydration, and movement:** These three indicators are essential parameters for your long-term health and weight management.
- Track how many hours you sleep. This may also motivate you to put healthier boundaries around time for rest.
- Measure how much water you drink every day—you will likely find yourself driven to increase your fluid intake.
- Notice your energy and enjoyment of moving your body.
- **Digestion and bowel movements:** Physical comfort after meals and having regular (ideally daily) bowel movements are key indicators of how your body is assimilating what you are feeding it. Keeping conscious of these factors enables you to adjust your diet to improve digestion, increasing or decreasing dietary fiber in response.
- **Skin, hair, and nails:** Notice how your diet may impact your complexion or the condition of your hair and nails.
- **Energy:** What we eat should support energy rather than drain us, giving us a reasonable amount of energy to live our lives. Energy levels and fatigue indicate whether we are eating the right amount of food and the right quality of food to meet our energy needs.

- **Periodic blood tests:** These routine tests and the general health assessment exam remain the best screening method to check your health status. They are also essential because they can reveal the existence of common diseases such as anemia, diabetes, blood clotting disorders, hepatitis, kidney failure, cardiovascular disease, and digestive or urinary tract infections.

MEASURING PROGRESS WITH YOUR RELATIONSHIP WITH FOOD

The following are all indicators of our relationship with food, and we can expect all of them to vary and fluctuate depending where we are and what is going on in our lives. Using them as prompts for reflection, return to them and ask yourself how true the statements feel for you. Remember, this is about self-awareness from a position of curiosity, not from a stance of self-judgment:

- Hunger cues: I am able to recognize and respond to my hunger cues.
- Satiety: I allow myself to eat to the point of satisfaction versus undereating or overeating.
- Pleasure around eating: I enjoy thinking about and eating whole foods and fun foods and treats.
- Inclusion: I eat all foods; I only restrict specific foods or groups of food if there is a medically valid reason.
- Body neutrality: I have a balanced view of my body. I err away from hyperfocus and strong feelings about my body, both positive and negative.
- Objectivity about scale: I think of the number on the scale as data rather than an assessment of my value.
- Unemotional eating: I can recognize emotional impulses to eat and distinguish these from hunger cues, in terms of both timing and what I want to eat.
- Obsessions and rigidity: I am able to recognize increases in obsessive and/or rigid thoughts or behaviors about food and my body. I understand that these are signals of personal stress and strain that need my attention.

- Food association: I do not associate certain foods with being unhealthy. I understand certain foods are more calorie dense and therefore should be consumed in smaller quantities.
- Perfectionism: I am able to move away from the idea that there is a perfect way to eat or perfect body.

APPENDIX F

MACROS MINIMALLY PROCESSED WHOLE FOODS LIST

CARBOHYDRATES

Whole-grain breads

Rice

Oats

Buckwheat

Whole-grain pasta

Potatoes

Sweet potatoes

Pumpkin

Squashes

Fruits

Vegetables

CARBOHYDRATE/PROTEIN

Beans: chickpeas, black beans, black-eyed peas, cannellini beans, lima beans, pinto beans, peas, kidney beans

Lentils

Quinoa

Fruit yogurts

Milk

Peas

PROTEIN

Beef: tenderloin, T-bone, top sirloin, lean ground beef

Chicken: skinless breast, skinless thighs, lean ground chicken

Turkey: skinless breast, skinless thighs, lean ground turkey

Lamb

White fish

Cottage cheese, low-fat, no-fat

Plain yogurts

Egg whites

Protein powder

Tofu

Tempeh

PROTEIN/FATS

Eggs

Salmon

Meat, high-fat cuts of meat: filet mignon, T-bone, New York strip, porterhouse, flap or skirt steak, and rib-eye steaks

Chicken, dark meat

Turkey, dark meat

Milk, full fat

Cottage cheese, full fat

FATS

Nut butters

Nuts: almonds, cashews, macadamia, hazelnuts, pecans

Seeds: chia seeds, flaxseeds, hemp seeds, sesame seeds, pumpkin seeds, sunflower seeds

Avocado

Vegetable oils: extra-virgin olive oil, avocado oil, flaxseed oil, sesame oil, coconut oil

Egg yolks

Flax seeds

Olives

Chia Seeds

APPENDIX G

WORKING WITH A NUTRITION EXPERT

When using the macros framework to maintain, lose, or gain weight, it can be helpful for anyone to work with a nutritionist, dietician, or food coach for a period of time.

Getting help from an expert is a logical decision that will save you time, simplify the process, and help you achieve sustainable results.

A dietician, nutritionist, or food coach can help you:

- navigate complex nutritional information and simplify food decisions,
- create a personalized meal plan,
- make food choices that lead to the results you want, and
- stay on track for lifetime weight management.

Specific to following a macros eating pattern, a dietician, nutritionist, and food coach helps to:

- set appropriate and realistic targets,
- calculate the number of calories you need to eat to reach your goals,
- calculate your macros percentages,
- clarify how long to be in a calorie deficit or surplus,
- guide you through the reverse dieting phase,
- instruct you on how to maintain your weight after reaching a realistic weight goal for your height and age,
- discover nutritional deficiencies—you may have a deficiency of vitamins, a deficiency of minerals, or you may not eat enough protein,

- permanently guide you through the process and offer the needed support, and
- give you tools to reach your goals and teach you how to implement them on your own.

They can help you stop:

- extreme approaches to eating and wellness, and
- spending hours and hours thinking and worrying about food and/or your body.

HOW TO CHOOSE A NUTRITION EXPERT

Hiring a nutrition expert can feel confusing because it is somewhat of a saturated market. When sifting through the Google search results and social media posts to find an expert who is the right fit for you, pay attention to these things:

- **Credentials:** Higher education is essential. Research produces new insights all the time, so coaches should be constantly learning, updating, and expanding their knowledge. If you have a specific health issue, look for a coach with the specific credentials.
- **Resources:** A nutrition expert will share resources to teach you to eat better, such as recipes, meal plans, eating tips for your lifestyle, and tips for eating out.
- **Data:** Nutrition, health, and weight loss are scientific, and your coach should request data from you on a regular basis in order to track your progress and make adjustments in response. This data will include things like food logs, measurements including body weight, and information about sleep and mood.
- **Specialism:** A nutrition coach cannot and should not diagnose medical conditions. However, they can support the management of diagnosed conditions by recommending lifestyle and nutrition changes to minimize symptoms and improve quality of life.
- **Support:** A coach should inspire you and celebrate your efforts to create a healthier lifestyle. Sharing your thoughts and feelings about your body and food is essential, and your coach's non-judgmental attitude will support progress.

- **Referral:** If a friend refers you to a coach, ask them to describe their experience. Asking questions about the coach in particular and what accountability was present will give you a sense of what you will be receiving.
- **Style:** Every coach has a different style, and shopping around to find one that works for you isn't a bad thing. Ask for a meeting prior to signing up to ensure their style is a good fit for you.
- **Realism:** A coach should support your progress toward achievable and healthy weight and exercise goals. If you have an unhealthy weight goal or an unrealistic timeline in mind to reach your goal, a coach should help you redefine healthy goals.

ACKNOWLEDGMENTS

Thank you to the Turner Publishing team for saying yes to *Kosher Macros* and improving the manuscript!

I consulted with nutrition experts for this project to ensure the accuracy of technical information shared in these pages. Their knowledge and training improved the technical information included, especially in the annexes. Thank you to Optimal Wellness Nutrition coaching experts Alyssa Wheelis, Hanna Hawkins and Nicole Fieber. Thank you to RD Nutrition and Wellness founder Julie McGee.

To Bonny Coombe, our positive and productive working relationship and style is something I feel proud of. Speaking with you on a regular basis is intellectually stimulating and therapeutic (in part because you make me laugh so much). You are shining and achieving with Lakhon Komnit ("thinking theater" in Khmer) in Cambodia, through your hard work and dedication!

Thank you to recipe testers from the Jewish Food Hero newsletter. Your feedback was encouraging and helpful to making selected recipes better!

To my mother and father, for their unconditional love and support. Since moving away from veganism, it's been so comforting to be able to enjoy my mother's food again.

À Charles, merci d'être ouvert aux nouvelles idées et aux nouvelles recettes. Vivre en France a rendu tes idées sur la nourriture plus réelles: le plaisir et la modération sont de mise.

Yaël, eating everything (kosher) with you, and seeing you enjoy all foods in moderation, has to me been the most rewarding part of the change forward from veganism. I was so happy for you when you finally tried kosher McDonald's in the Israel airport in May 2022. Our ritual of mini ice-cream cones as a treat is a highlight for me! New motto: K.Y.P.S.

Je t'aime.

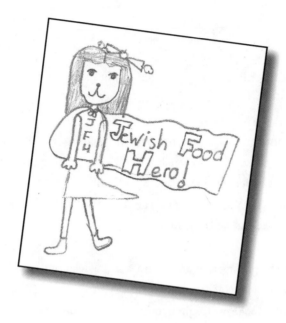

The Jewish Food Hero by Yaël Alfond-Vincent

GOING FORWARD

If I left out your favorite recipe, I am sorry. There are so many recipes that could have been in this book, and I wish I could have included everyone's favorites.

Going forward, I will be continuing my efforts to develop Jewish Food Hero. I would appreciate your help with this. Please write me an email at kenden@jewishfoodhero.com and tell me your suggestions for Jewish Food Hero and your favorite recipes so I can try to include them in a future project.

INDEX

ABOUT THE AUTHOR

Kenden Alfond is a psychotherapist based in Paris, France, where she lives with her husband and daughter. In 2005 she was an American Jewish World Service volunteer in India and went on to use her expertise in psychology in clinical and humanitarian work in Afghanistan, DR Congo, Switzerland, and Cambodia. She started Jewish Food Hero in 2015 to get healthier plant-based and vegan food onto Jewish tables around the world. Through her organization, Kenden strives to improve our mental, emotional, and physical health and help the environment. Kenden holds a BA in Literature from Brown University and an MA in Counseling Psychology from Naropa University.